VITAL LIFE

Secrets to Stay Young and Live Longer

REVOLUTIONARY PLAN TO REVERSE BIOLOGICAL AGE
AND MODIFY GENETIC BLUEPRINT

VITAL LIFE

Increase Your Energy, Strength, Cognition & Performance

Secrets to Stay Young and Live Longer

Proven Program of Twenty Years Using Cutting-Edge
Regenerative Anti-aging Therapies to Reclaim
Youthful Vitality and Reverse Diseases

HARDESH GARG, MD

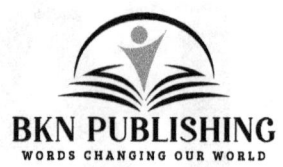

BKN PUBLISHING
WORDS CHANGING OUR WORLD

Copyright © 2025 by Hardesh Garg, MD

All rights reserved

No portion of this book may be reproduced, stored in a retrieval system, or transmitted in any form by any means—electronic, mechanical, photocopy, recording, or other—except for brief quotations in printed reviews, without prior permission of the author.

Hardcover ISBN: 9798998629105
Paperback ISBN: 9798998629112
eBook ISBN: 9798998629129

DISCLAIMER

To protect privacy and maintain confidentiality, the names of individuals mentioned in this book have been changed.

The content of this book reflects the opinions and insights of the author and is intended to provide helpful and informative material on the topics discussed. This book is sold with the understanding that the author, publisher, and all others involved in its creation are not providing medical, health, or other professional services. Readers are strongly advised to consult their physician, healthcare provider, or another qualified medical professional before adopting any recommendations or drawing conclusions based on the information presented.

Throughout this book, the author may discuss various companies and entities in which the author has no financial interest.

The author and publisher explicitly disclaim all responsibility for any liability, loss, risk, or harm—personal or otherwise—that may result, directly or indirectly, from the use or application of the material in this book.

SOCIAL IMPACT

A portion of the profits from this book will be donated to these nonprofit organizations working hard to help people with healthcare, mental wellness, and hunger in America: Project Hope, the National Alliance on Mental Illness (NAMI), and Feeding America.

DEDICATION

To my parents in heaven, who sacrificed so much and encouraged me relentlessly in my journey to become a physician despite countless adversities. To my wonderful wife, an angel who loves me unconditionally, even in moments when I do not deserve it. To my two incredible sons, who fill my heart with gratitude and remind me daily of the infinite blessings of the Almighty Consciousness. And to my brothers and sisters in healthcare, who dedicate themselves tirelessly to healing and serving humanity.

CONTENTS

Preface — XI

Part 1. Introduction to a Youthful Rejuvenation
- Chapter 1. Invitation: A Journey to Youthful Longevity — 1
- Chapter 2. Off the Beaten Path — 12
- Chapter 3. The Eternal Search for the Fountain of Youth — 22
- Chapter 4. The VitalLife Program: An Overview — 33

Part 2. Understanding the Science of Aging
- Chapter 5. Unraveling the Mysteries of Aging: The Science of Why We Age — 47
- Chapter 6. A Disease Called Aging — 65

Part 3. The VitalLife Program for a Younger and Vibrant You
- Chapter 7. A Personalized Assessment: Biomarkers and DNA Tests — 87
- Chapter 8. Unleashing the Power of Regenerative Medicine: Turning Back the Clock — 97
- Chapter 9. Stem Cells and Exosomes: Stimulating Cellular Regeneration — 114
- Chapter 10. Psychedelics in Rejuvenation and Healing — 137
- Chapter 11. Optimizing Hormones and Peptides for Youthful Vitality — 169
- Chapter 12. Mastering Metabolism: Mitochondrial Dysfunction and Insulin Resistance — 188
- Chapter 13. Fighting Systemic Chronic Inflammation: Boosting Immune and Gut Health — 204
- Chapter 14. Ultra-Personalized Compounded Medications — 222

Part 4. Lifestyle Changes for Endless Youthfulness

Chapter 15.	Embracing a Plant-Based Diet: Improve Life and Longevity	243
Chapter 16.	Exercise for Strength and Vitality	281
Chapter 17.	Supplements and Herbs: Secrets of Nature's Remedies	291
Chapter 18.	The Power of Mindfulness and Restful Sleep: A Stress-Free, Energetic Life	299

Part 5. Conclusion: A Journey of Rejuvenation

Chapter 19.	Your 6-Step Action Plan for Youthfulness and Longevity	319
Chapter 20.	Embracing a Brand-New You	331

Acknowledgments	337
Practical Resources for Improved Healthspan and Longevity	341
Index	355
About the Author	371

PREFACE

Our bodies possess an extraordinary, innate power to regenerate, heal, and thrive —regardless of our age. Within these pages lies your blueprint for unlocking incredible potential you may not yet realize you have.

I believe strongly that it isn't just about living longer; it's about living better, more fully, more joyfully. With this blueprint, you can achieve that.

For the past four decades, I've dedicated my life to medicine, with the last twenty years focused on cutting-edge regenerative and longevity medicine. Through treating thousands of patients from all walks of life with the latest breakthroughs in anti-aging and regenerative medicine, I've written *VitalLife* with a heartfelt purpose: to empower you with the knowledge and insights needed to transform your health and your life. This book is born not only from my extensive experience as a physician but also from a lifetime of bridging the cutting-edge advancements of Western medicine with the enduring wisdom of Eastern traditions.

Unlike traditional treatments that merely mask symptoms, VitalLife program goes beyond the surface, optimizing your body's biological functions to slow and repair cellular decline, fostering holistic and lasting rejuvenation from within. It not only enhances physical health and longevity but also aims to harmonize the mind, body, and soul, fostering emotional resilience and inner richness.

After all, what is the value of an extended life if our hearts are not whole and our spirits remain unfulfilled?

While I could have written a dense, scientific document brimming with research articles and references, I chose instead to write something far more practical and meaningful: a guide accessible to anyone seeking true youthfulness, cure from diseases, and longevity at any age. This is my life's work, offered as a road map, to help others discover their own path to more vibrant, healthier living. With this book, my mission is to democratize and popularize these distinctive therapies, once secrets of the wealthy and famous, and make them accessible to everyone.

My sincere hope is that the knowledge and insights you will gain throughout this book prepare you to make the choices that will dramatically improve the quality of your life. Whether you are in your thirties, fifties, or even seventies, your body is ready to respond to the changes you make today. I've seen patients who once thought they were too old or too far along in their disease turn their lives around completely. With a few targeted, consistent efforts, you will not only reclaim your lasting health, but also find a new sense of purpose and zest for life.

I want to inspire you to take charge of your health and embrace these transformative, unconventional approaches to youthfulness, optimal health, and reversing disease. And, to enjoy a longer life, lived better. Together we are shaping a future where the goal of lifelong youthfulness and living till an age of 150 or beyond will be not just a dream but an attainable reality for all.

PART 1
INTRODUCTION TO A YOUTHFUL REJUVENATION

CHAPTER 1

Invitation: A Journey to Youthful Longevity

> The good physician treats the disease; the great physician treats the patient who has the disease.
> —*Sir William Osler, esteemed Canadian physician (1849–1919)*

> A healthy man wants a thousand things;
> a sick man only wants one.
> —*Confucius, Chinese philosopher (551–479 BC)*

Just a few years ago, when Phil walked into my office, frustration and defeat were written all over his face. He was twenty pounds overweight, exhausted constantly, and plagued by brain fog and muscle aches. Though he was only forty-six years old, his once-strong muscles felt weaker by the day, and although he was a professional golfer on the PGA Tour, now his body seemed to betray him. He was disciplined, eating a high-protein, low-carbohydrate diet, taking a cocktail of supplements, and hitting the gym three to four times a week. Yet nothing seemed to work.

In addition to seeing his family physician, Phil had consulted with several specialists, including a cardiologist, an endocrinologist, and a neurologist. His doctors had given him the usual advice: eat more vegetables, exercise more, and lose weight. But Phil knew deep down something was wrong. "It feels like my body has just shut down," he told me, disheartened. He had resigned himself to believing this was the inevitable price of aging. By the time he saw me, he was losing hope in his professional career and convinced his best days were behind him.

Phil's lab results painted a clearer picture. Not only was he overweight and struggling mentally and physically, but his cholesterol was high, he was prediabetic, and his blood pressure had crept into the danger zone. Surprisingly, his level of testosterone, the primary male sex hormone, was as high as an eighteen-year-old's—a clear sign that low testosterone wasn't the culprit, as it is for so many men his age.

What Phil needed wasn't generic advice or cookie-cutter solutions. I started him on a customized program incorporating specific regenerating products, special peptides, a personalized nutritional plan, and custom pharmacy compounds, along with targeted resistance training. Within six weeks, Phil's transformation was undeniable. His energy returned, his stamina soared, and he began to build muscle while shedding fat. The smile he thought he'd lost reappeared, especially when he stepped back onto the golf course with a renewed sense of purpose.

Phil realized what so many others need to hear: the struggles he faced weren't an unavoidable part of aging. With the right approach, he reclaimed not just his career but also his hope and vitality.

Throughout my medical career of over forty years, countless patients have asked one question that cuts straight to the heart of human vulnerability. It comes not just from my patients but also from family and friends—people who trust me with their deepest fears about their health and aging. Sure, they ask about longevity and stem cells, but what really echoes in these conversations are words tinged with confusion and often despair: "Doc, I'm so young; then why do I feel so old?" or "Doc, why do I feel so drained all the time despite being so young?" The frustration in their voices and the look in their eyes—it tells a story of disconnect between their inner spirit and their physical reality. While most men and women asking such questions are in their fifties or older, I'm hearing them increasingly from people in their forties—and even younger—who convey a mix of disbelief and discontent.

What experience has taught me is profound: while the desire to live longer is universal, there is something far more urgent in people's hearts. Since ancient times, human beings have been searching for that mythical fountain of *youth* and not so much a fountain of *immortality*. They're all seeking that fire, that spark of vitality that makes each day worth living. They're not just chasing numbers on a calendar; they're really after that youthful energy to pursue their dreams, the stamina to perform at their peak, and that indefinable sense of well-being that makes life rich, jubilant, and meaningful at any age. They're yearning for a life where every moment pulses with zest, where joy isn't rationed, where fulfillment isn't something reserved for their memories.

At sixty-three, I don't just understand these feelings—I live them. Sure, the prospect of a longer life is appealing to me, but, like you, what sets my soul on fire is the desire to stay vibrantly healthy and spend my remaining years immersed in what brings me joy: living each day with purpose, my heart full of gratitude, and finding meaning in serving others. I share the same fears as my fellow baby boomers and Gen Xers: we've watched our parents' generation shuffle between medical appointments and hospitals, their lives gradually shrinking into a routine of pill bottles, doctor visits, and daily limitations.

That's not the future any of us envision. We don't want our world to contract, to give up the simple but profound pleasures that make life worth living, whether it's the exhilaration of hiking a challenging trail, the wonder of exploring new places, or the precious moments with children and grandchildren that no medicine can replace.

Throughout my years in medicine, I've witnessed something that still fills me with awe: the treatments I use don't just extend life's timeline—they reignite its very essence. Nothing moves me more deeply than watching someone rediscover their vitality through my regenerative and anti-aging protocols. Whether they're battling the grinding weight of chronic pain, the worry of heart disease, the limitations of arthritis, the frustration of brain fog, or just that pervasive feeling of being "old"—seeing their transformation is like watching spring return after a long winter.

That profound impact is what drove me to write this book. After my years of clinical experience, I want to share these breakthrough technologies not just as medical protocols, but as keys to unlock renewed possibility in your life. This journey we're embarking on isn't simply about longevity—it's about rekindling that inner fire, that youthful essence that makes every day an adventure worth living.

My Journey to a New World

Though it was more than thirty-five years ago, I remember it as if it happened yesterday. It was a hot and sweaty summer morning in 1989, and I was standing outside my home in the bustling city of New Delhi, India. At twenty-eight, I held two treasures: my medical degree and an American dream. The air was thick with memories—morning chants mixing with the aroma of healing herbs, wisdom passed down through generations echoing in my grandmother's Ayurvedic remedies, and the profound understanding that healing was never just about the body but also about the spirit that animated it. These weren't just cultural touchstones; they were the very fabric of my being, woven through years of watching people heal through a harmonious dance of ancient wisdom and community love.

My medical training took place at a prestigious institution in New Delhi, one of the top medical colleges in India. We were immersed in the principles of Western medicine, and our education and training closely mirrored that of American medical schools. However, at the time, the Indian healthcare system lagged behind the US system by at least two decades, with a stark difference in the availability of innovative treatments, latest medicines, advanced technologies, modern imaging, and hospital infrastructure. This gap between what we learned in medical school and what we could apply to help our patients was a constant source of frustration, but it also taught us resilience and resourcefulness.

What set our experience apart was the holistic approach to health that was deeply ingrained in both daily life and clinical practice. This wasn't something taught in textbooks, but rather an intrinsic part of Indian culture. Yoga, meditation, and spirituality were as essential to health as the medicines we prescribed. Food was considered medicine, with freshly cooked meals rich in Indian herbs and spices, abundant fruits and vegetables the norm, augmented by natural supplements if necessary. Family love, strong community connections, and vibrant social lives added emotional and healing dimensions to well-being that extended far beyond clinical care.

For many physicians, including myself, coming to America was a dream—a chance to build a better future and immerse ourselves in the cutting-edge advancements of the US medical system. The opportunity to learn and practice state-of-the-art treatments and technologies, access to the latest clinical research, and the prime healthcare delivery system were irresistible prospects. Yet I carried with me the holistic values and traditions that had shaped my early years, a combination of perspectives that would deeply influence my approach to medicine.

When I boarded that flight to America a couple of weeks later, my heart thundered with equal measures of anticipation and anxiety. Was I leaving behind not just my homeland but also a whole philosophy of healing and cultural norms and mores? Yet, the allure of the American lifestyle, coupled with the opportunity to learn the latest scientific approaches and practice modern medicine in the United States pulled me forward like a powerful magnet. The young doctor in me burned with ambition and curiosity. What wonders would America and its latest Western medicine reveal?

A few years later, landing the assistant professor position at the University of Florida College of Medicine felt like achieving an important milestone. Those early days sparkled with possibilities: the thrill of clinical research, the joy of watching young doctors' eyes light up with understanding, the satisfaction of teaching nurses and other healthcare providers who shared my passion for healing. I was living my dream, or so I thought.

Beneath the surface, something began to stir. A quiet voice, at first barely a whisper, grew louder with each passing day. As I wrote prescription after prescription, ordered test after test, I felt myself becoming a mere technician of symptoms rather than a healer of people. The patients I saw weren't just cases of diabetes, obesity, heart conditions, or arthritis—they were human beings whose spirits dimmed with each new complication, whose hopes faded with each additional medication.

The disillusionment crept in slowly, then all at once. Here I was, practicing and teaching medicine at a prestigious institution, yet feeling increasingly hollow. *We were always too late*—waiting for diseases to manifest, watching helplessly as complications mounted. And the contrast with my early experiences in India, where healing was preventive and holistic, became painfully stark.

I knew deep in my soul that there had to be a better way. Medicine, as I had been practicing and observing it, seemed incomplete, focused too often on merely suppressing symptoms rather than addressing the whole person. I felt it in every fiber of my being: the future of medicine must go beyond treating isolated ailments. It must embrace holistic healing, where the mind, body, and spirit work together in harmony.

As a physician, I believed that true healing entailed not always necessarily curing a condition but restoring balance, comfort, and dignity. I longed for a practice where I could offer healing, even in moments when a cure was beyond reach—where I could ease suffering and empower patients to reclaim their vitality. This yearning shaped my journey going forward, guiding me toward a more integrated, compassionate approach to care.

In the fall of 2004, I made a decision that my colleagues thought was madness: leaving my comfortable academic position to start something revolutionary. Medisolare wasn't just a clinic; it was my vision of healing come to life, a bridge between worlds. The name itself—combining medicine and sun—reflected my deep belief that healing comes from both scientific innovation and nature's wisdom. At Medisolare, to provide comprehensive holistic care, my team included an herbalist, a yoga teacher, a nutritionist, a mindfulness expert, and an acupuncturist.

This wasn't just a professional pivot; it was a return to my roots while reaching for the future. The memories of my childhood in India, where its traditional system of medicine, *Ayurveda*, along with yoga and meditation, were as natural as breathing, merged with my years of Western medical training. The VitalLife program arose from this fusion—not as another superficial "anti-aging" program pushing quick fixes, but as a comprehensive journey toward genuine wellness.

What happened next still fills me with awe. People began coming to Medisolare not just from across America but from around the globe. Each carried their own story of disillusionment with traditional medicine—the athletes struggling with chronic pain, the executives feeling decades older than their age, the celebrities trying to maintain their beauty without surgery, the grandmother wanting to dance at her grandchild's wedding. Their trust in me, their willingness to try a different path, touched me deeply.

The transformations I witnessed became my greatest joy and deepest source of fulfillment. Each success story reinforced the power of a comprehensive, personalized, and data-driven approach to healing. With the VitalLife program, I wasn't just helping patients with youthfulness—I was empowering them to reverse diseases, and enjoy healthier, more vibrant lives for longer.

For me, as for so many of you, it's more about being in the best shape of your life, no matter your age, and rediscovering the youthfulness you thought was lost forever. Watching someone rediscover their vitality, seeing the sparkle return to their eyes, hearing them say, "I feel twenty years younger"—these moments filled my heart with an indescribable mixture of happiness and gratitude. Professional athletes from the National Football League, the PGA Tour, and the Association of Tennis Professionals (ATP) found their way to us, seeking not just performance enhancement but also true healing. Yet it was the everyday victories that moved me most: the diabetic patient reducing her medications, the arthritis sufferer regaining mobility, the exhausted soul reclaiming his zest for life.

Over these past two decades, my understanding of healing has sculpted its own path—like a river, slowly yet persistently, carving and shaping a stone, revealing deeper truths with each passing year. I became more and more convinced of the *inner healing power of our bodies*, when given the proper environment to thrive and flourish. The human body's capacity for renewal is nothing short of miraculous, a symphony of regeneration waiting for the right conductor. Through careful orchestration—blending cutting-edge stem cell treatments with precisely calibrated hormone optimization, thoughtfully targeted supplements, and profound lifestyle transformations—while staying true to the timeless wisdom of nutrition, acupuncture, yoga, and mindfulness, I found myself creating something that transcended ordinary medicine.

> When provided with the right environment, our bodies possess an extraordinary innate power to regenerate, heal, and thrive—regardless of our age.

For the first time in my journey as a healer, I felt complete alignment with my calling. Each day brought new confirmations that this approach was the path forward. Moreover, I was feeling purposeful and blissful and thankful to that one infinite consciousness. The soulful vibrations that I'd experienced during those early-morning meditations in Delhi were now manifesting themselves in the healing journeys of my patients.

When the COVID pandemic forced the world to pause beginning in early 2020, I found my moment to share this knowledge more broadly through writing this book. I share not only protocols and treatments but also a vision of healing that honors both the scientific and the sacred, the measurable and the age-old. This is my life's work, offered to you to help you shape your own journey to a vibrant, meaningful living—a journey that I began tracing long ago in the streets of Delhi and now continue to walk each day with profound gratitude and joy.

A Personal Invitation for a Journey to Your Best Self

Over the years, I've crafted the VitalLife program as a living, breathing lifestyle that marries tomorrow's biohacking innovations with from patient-centered approaches such as *holistic medicine* and *functional medicine*. (Briefly, holistic medicine takes into account the whole person, including their physical, mental, emotional, social, and spiritual health, while functional medicine focuses on treating the root causes of disease rather than just the symptoms.) *As the science evolved, so did this program. I still continue to update it with new medical discoveries and proven, safe technologies.*

As a physician who has seen both the successes and shortcomings of our healthcare system, I want to share with you a deeply personal perspective. My own battle with chronic fatigue syndrome—possibly brought on by post-COVID inflammation—was both humbling and eye-opening, providing a heartfelt firsthand experience as a patient of our traditional healthcare system's limitations. I have witnessed the suffering of my angelic wife of thirty-six years from schizophrenia, as well as several close family members afflicted with chronic diseases and serious brain illnesses, despite having followed all the "right" advice from conventional medical standards. This, coupled with the concussion my wife experienced in early 2017, changed my life and career trajectory. Today I am totally devoted to finding a cure for the progressive and debilitating diseases of aging, especially brain illnesses. Through my personal health challenges, my family's experiences, and witnessing those life-changing benefits for my patients, I've observed the transformative power of the VitalLife program. I'm not speaking in hypotheticals or possibilities—I'm referring to the science that has transformed countless lives. The future of aging isn't about passive acceptance but about creating tangible, positive changes.

As I continue my work in regenerative and anti-aging medicine, I'm increasingly optimistic about the future of its preventive and therapeutic possibilities. The potential to enhance cellular regeneration, optimize metabolic function, and improve physiological resilience through these interventions is unprecedented. We're approaching an era where targeted regenerative protocols, which I will explain in depth, can effectively address conditions ranging from metabolic dysfunction, to cognitive decline, to age-related degeneration. This is precisely why I became passionate about this specialized field over two decades ago, dedicating my career to advancing the clinical applications of regenerative and anti-aging medicine.

Consider this book my personal invitation to you to reimagine what's possible. You can now forget the notion that your best self is in the past—I'm here to show you it's just around the corner. By harnessing the latest breakthroughs in anti-aging and regenerative medicine, we'll explore how to rebuild your body from the cellular level up, fostering profound and lasting health. And here's something even more exciting: the strategies outlined in this book don't just affect a single condition, such as heart disease or stroke, but promote healing and thwart disease progression throughout your entire body.

The strategies described in this program have been used successfully by so many of my patients over the years. You'll meet a number of them here, sharing their stories. People like Phil, who had been under the care of numerous physicians and specialists, receiving traditional treatments for various diagnoses but with little success.

What's truly remarkable is that many of these life-changing strategies, especially when adopted in your twenties or thirties, can be as straightforward as making simple changes to your diet and lifestyle. Even if you've already started experiencing symptoms of aging or have been diagnosed with a disease, it is still possible to halt its progression—and even reverse it.

At times, some of the information in this book might seem overwhelming or even repetitive, but I assure you, every detail serves a meaningful purpose. Each piece is included to address the who, what, where, why, and how of the VitalLife program, enabling you to effectively apply the insights contained in these pages to your own health journey.

For me, it's truly a privilege to practice medicine in an era of such profound scientific advancement. As we look to the future, I'm more convinced than ever that we're just beginning to unlock the full potential of science of living longer, healthier.

Before we delve into the science of aging and the specifics of VitalLife, let's first explore some fundamental health and wellness concepts in chapter 2. Understanding these will help you grasp why the VitalLife approach to longevity and youthfulness often diverges from traditional Western medicine—and why that's exactly what makes it so effective.

CHAPTER 2

Off the Beaten Path

...For what is a man, what has he got?
If not himself, then he has naught
To say the things he truly feels
And not the words of one who kneels
The record shows I took the blows
And did it my way
...Yes, it was my way.
—*"My Way", Sung by Frank Albert Sinatra, American singer and actor (1915–1998)*

Two roads diverged in a wood and I—I took the
one less traveled by,
and that has made all the difference.
—*"The Road Not Taken," Robert Frost,
American poet (1874–1963)*

I believe I was born with a fondness—or as some would call it, a weakness—for not accepting dogmas, traditions, and conventions without first asking "Why?" Perhaps that's why my spirit has always resonated with Robert Frost's "The Road Not Taken" and Frank Sinatra's iconic rendition of "My Way," which quite earnestly, for me embody the American anthem of self-determination, striking a deep chord within my being. I felt especially compelled to question traditions that led to less-than-ideal outcomes, whether for the many or even just a few. Admittedly, this habit landed me in more than a few sticky situations—whether with elders in India or with a few of those self-proclaimed intellectuals in ivory towers—but over time it has served me well. This same curiosity and refusal to accept the status quo is what ultimately inspired me to challenge traditional medicine and design the VitalLife program in order to have a significant impact on health and disease.

As a physician dedicated to optimizing human health and preventing and curing diseases, in this chapter I want to first explore with you the silent progression of declining health and chronic diseases. Through my personal and clinical experiences, I've witnessed both the strengths and shortcomings of our traditional Western healthcare system—a system familiar to us all. In this chapter, we'll also explore the challenges within our traditional Western system of healthcare, particularly when it comes to preventing and reversing diseases.

Before we venture off the beaten path of conventional care, it's crucial that we discuss several key concepts that will frame our discussion. The distinction between *healthspan* and *lifespan* is fundamental, as is the important difference between *biological age* and *chronological age*. These concepts have revolutionized how I approach patient care.

Based on these key concepts, the VitalLife program is developed to deviate from conventional medical paradigms. These concepts, while not typically emphasized in traditional medical training, have profound implications for health optimization, disease prevention and management, as well as for youthful longevity. I've constantly observed in my practice how understanding these key processes can dramatically alter the trajectory of chronic disease development, often before conventional medicine would even recognize a problem.

As we venture beyond traditional care, understanding these mechanisms becomes crucial for implementing more effective, proactive interventions. Let us explore some of these concepts in greater detail.

The Silent Progression of Chronic Diseases: Understanding the Hidden Timeline

The cellular and molecular science of development of chronic diseases reveals one of medicine's most crucial insights: by the time symptoms emerge, the underlying pathological processes have often been developing for decades.

The number one killer in United States, cardiovascular disease, presents a compelling example of this silent progression. What's particularly striking is how atherosclerosis (arterial blockages) begins appearing in the arteries' interior walls *as early as the teenage years*, yet clinical symptoms typically don't emerge until the fifth or sixth decade. Advanced imaging studies reveal fatty streaks and early plaque formation in young adults who appear otherwise completely healthy. These early changes progress gradually over decades before manifesting as angina, heart attack, or stroke.

The same pattern emerges across multiple chronic conditions. Type 2 diabetes often develops silently for five to ten years or even longer before it's diagnosed by traditional tests, with insulin resistance and metabolic dysfunction establishing long before blood sugar levels become clinically significant.

> By the time symptoms emerge, the underlying pathological processes have been developing for years, even decades.

Similarly, neurodegenerative processes such as Alzheimer's disease begin decades before cognitive symptoms appear. Research demonstrates that damaging amyloid protein accumulation and neuroinflammatory changes can start twenty to thirty years before clinical manifestation. This understanding fundamentally shifts our approach from treating symptoms to identifying and addressing these processes in their earliest stages.

This recognition of disease progression's timeline underscores a fundamental truth in medicine: *prevention proves far more effective than treatment.* From my years of experience, I can tell you with certainty that by understanding and addressing these underlying processes early, we can markedly alter these disease trajectories before they become clinically significant.

Where Traditional Medicine Falls Short

Let me share something that still makes me disheartened with my medical profession—a truth I have witnessed as a physician and after my own family's health challenges that breaks my heart. Most of us grew up trusting traditional Western medicine, and, yes, it works miracles in emergencies and through surgeries. *But there's a profound flaw at its core that I can no longer stay quiet about.* Imagine a house with a cracking foundation. Instead of fixing the cracks, we're just painting over them, again and again. That's what modern healthcare has become: a sophisticated system of masking symptoms while the underlying problems grow silently.

I see it in the tired eyes of my family members and my patients. They've faithfully taken every prescription, followed every guideline, yet something essential is missing. Traditional healthcare has become like a game of whack-a-mole: symptoms pop up, we suppress them with medications, only to have new ones surface elsewhere. *We're not healing, we're just managing decline.* You see, physicians are trained to find and treat diseases; they are not trained to do anything for your healing and wellness. And, sadly, so many of them are focused mostly on diseases and not so much on the patient. We all know that, far too often, by the time a person is diagnosed with a chronic disease such as diabetes, hypertension, heart disease, or stroke, *it is already too late.*

I'll give you an example: a patient discovers his cholesterol or blood pressure is high. He's prescribed a medication, and yes, his numbers improve on paper. But nobody asks the crucial question: Why are his arteries struggling in the first place? Another patient's blood sugar spikes, and she's given diabetes medication. Her numbers stabilize, but her body's underlying inability to utilize the hormone *insulin* efficiently continues unaddressed, like a car engine misfiring while we simply turn up the radio to mask the sound. I see this happen far too often with so many patients.

> Modern healthcare is a sophisticated symptom-masking system, with a "drug-for-symptom" approach. We're NOT healing, we're just managing decline.

In addition to this "drug-for-symptom" approach, another centerpiece of our traditional Western healthcare system is its intense focus on specialization. This means one specialist for each organ or body system: a *cardiologist* for the heart, a *pulmonologist* for the lungs, a *neurologist* for the brain, a *nephrologist* for the kidneys, and so on. While these specialists possess an extraordinary depth of knowledge about their respective organ system, they often lack a broader understanding of how the entire body functions as an interconnected system. And even more concerning, the person as a whole is frequently overlooked and gets mistreated.

The reality is that the body does not operate as a collection of isolated parts; it functions in unison as a cohesive, integrated whole. For example, signals from the gut greatly influence brain health, while those same signals impact the heart and lungs. This interconnectedness means that a problem in one organ can ripple across multiple systems, yet the current model of care tends to treat issues in silos. For many patients, this fragmented approach can be detrimental, as diseases and illnesses are rarely confined to just one organ.

Let me share a common scenario I'm certain you can relate to. It is happening every day in every town in this country. A patient receives a diagnosis of diabetes or coronary artery disease—conditions that, as we discussed, are frequently detected far too late in their disease progression. They diligently follow their doctor's recommendations: taking prescribed medications, adopting a healthier diet, incorporating supplements, increasing physical activity, and achieving weight loss. While their laboratory values may show improvement, I often see these patients soon cycling through various specialists for different disease complications.

For instance, they may find themselves consulting a cardiologist for heart angioplasty (a medical procedure to open up blocked or narrowed blood vessels supplying the heart muscle), a vascular surgeon for a blockage of the carotid artery in the neck, a neurologist for stroke prevention, a vascular surgeon again for peripheral arterial disease in the body's extremities, or a nephrologist for emerging kidney dysfunction. This cascade of specialist visits brings endless medications, laboratory tests, doctor appointments, and hospital stays.

Each specialist, with genuine dedication and expertise, focuses on managing complications AFTER they manifest in the respective organ system of his or her specialty. But here's what troubles me most: What about the root cause—*atherosclerosis*? This systemic disease process, causing arterial blockages throughout the entire body, often begins as early as in our twenties, sometimes even earlier. Surprisingly, we don't have specialists dedicated specifically to addressing this fundamental pathology.

Cardiologists often serve as proxies, but I've observed they're typically overwhelmed with performing angioplasties and prescribing cholesterol-reducing medications known as statins. They rarely have time to engage in crucial discussions about nutrition, exercise, targeted supplementation, or alternative therapeutic approaches. Most concerning is that patients are seldom informed about addressing the root cause of their health crisis—a solution that extends far beyond medication compliance and basic lifestyle modifications.

This drug-for-symptom approach with an intense focus on specialization has transformed healthcare into something that barely resembles *healthcare* at all. It has become a sophisticated system in which physicians are taught to expect decline and accept deterioration as inevitable. *Physicians measure success not by vibrant health but by how slowly we're losing ground.*

Every loss feels like a personal failure—a devastating indictment of the medical system I was trained to trust and once wholeheartedly believed in. As a physician, these experiences weigh heavily on my heart, leaving me grappling with the profound disconnect between what our system promises and what it delivers. They have forever changed me, pushing me to reimagine what true healing and compassionate care should look like.

This is why the VitalLife program was born from both frustration and hope. It's designed to fill this void in traditional medicine, offering something fundamentally different. Instead of just managing decline, the program activates your body's innate regenerative powers. We're not just treating symptoms—we're rewriting the story of how you age. I believe this what healthcare should strive to be: proactive, tailored to individual needs, and driven by the latest scientific breakthroughs.

Chronological Age versus Biological Age

Imagine two watches, crafted by the same artisan in the same year. One is meticulously cared for—its gears oiled, its mechanism calibrated with precision. The other is neglected, its parts grinding with every tick, its movements labored and strained. Though both display the same time, their inner workings reveal entirely different realities. One thrives, running with seamless precision, while the other struggles to keep pace.

Our bodies mirror this analogy. While we may share a birth year with others, the way we nurture ourselves shapes how our internal systems age. Chronological age simply counts the number of years you've lived, but biological age tells a far more revealing story: how old your body truly feels and functions.

It's fascinating, really. Haven't we all met someone who seems to defy aging? That energetic seventy-year-old who runs marathons while their couch-potato contemporary can barely climb stairs. That's biological age at work. It's like our body's own intimate diary, recording every healthy meal, every workout, every stressed-out day, every peaceful night's sleep.

Biological age is measured through physiological and molecular markers such as good and bad cholesterol, DNA tests, and inflammation blood tests, reflecting the health of your cells, tissues, and organs. It captures the cumulative effects of your lifestyle choices, genetics, and environment. This number is more than a statistic—it's a snapshot of how well you've maintained the intricate machinery of your body.

The good news is that our bodies are not static. With the right approach, we can recalibrate and rejuvenate, turning back the biological clock to restore health, vitality, and balance. What makes this particularly exciting is that *we're not just passive readers of our biological story—we can actually become its authors.*

If your biological age is higher than your calendar age, it's like getting an early warning system—a chance to make changes before small health issues become big ones. And if your biological age is lower? Well, that's your body's way of giving you a high five for taking good care of it.

I have spent years perfecting this science of health and biological age improvement. The comprehensive approach in VitalLife is like having a personal time machine for your cells. For example, through a combination of cutting-edge regenerative treatments—such as *senolytics* (think of them as your body's cleanup crew), *exosomes* (your body's chemical messengers for cellular healing), and *hormone optimization* (sending in the chemical repair team)—this program has shown that health and aging aren't just something that happens to us—they're something we can actively influence. Add to this the power of lifestyle modifications, proper sleep, and personalized medicine, and you've got *a powerful recipe for not just adding years to your life but adding life to your years.*

Healthspan versus Lifespan: Understanding the Difference

Simply stated, lifespan refers to the total length of time we live, while healthspan refers to the period of life spent in good health, free from chronic diseases and disabilities. In my experience, most of us prefer not just *adding years to our life (lifespan)*, but also about *adding life to our years (healthspan)*, where we feel vibrant, strong, and fully alive. While interconnected, these two metrics represent distinct aspects of the aging process. Modern medicine has significantly extended the average lifespan by preventing premature mortality from pathogenic diseases and acute trauma.

But here's what truly excites me as a practitioner: *healthspan optimization*. This means maximizing the duration of life free from chronic diseases and debilities. In my clinical experience, I've observed that extended lifespan without corresponding healthspan optimization often results in prolonged periods of physiological decline and may lead to plain misery. That's why I'm passionate about helping my patients understand that my primary objective isn't just lifespan extension but maximizing the period of optimal biological function.

Crucially, biological age and healthspan are entwined in an elegant dance—*enhancing biological age improves healthspan*. The scientific advances in this field are remarkable. We're making groundbreaking discoveries in biotechnologies and regenerative medicine that target fundamental aging mechanisms such as cellular senescence, chronic inflammation, mitochondrial dysfunction, and metabolic dysregulation. We're getting closer to closing this healthspan–lifespan gap—imagine maintaining robust cellular function and physiological resilience well into advanced age.

> Biological age and healthspan are closely tied together. The better your cells function, the healthier you become. While chronological aging is inevitable, accelerated biological aging isn't. So, you do have control over your biological age and, therefore, over your healthspan.

Whether you're in your fourth decade or your eighth decade, the objective is to optimize your biological age and cellular function, thus maximizing your healthspan—life spent without diseases and disability.

Real Healthcare: A New Approach

As a physician who has dedicated more than two decades to regenerative and anti-aging medicine, I've come to understand deeply that true healthcare must evolve beyond the traditional reactive model. My vision centers on three powerful pillars: *prevention, regeneration,* and *optimization.*

This isn't speculative medicine, a futuristic dream; it's happening in my clinical practice every day. Through precision diagnostics and data-driven regenerative protocols, I am helping patients reclaim control of their physiological destiny. The traditional paradigm that correlated aging with inevitable decline has been fundamentally challenged by this evidence-based approach to biological age and healthspan optimization.

Now armed with some new concepts in these biological processes, let us turn our attention to the eternal search for the mystical fountain of youth, from ancient times to the modern-day push to attain healthy and longer life. This quest has become more sophisticated and science-based, with a greater focus on understanding and manipulating the fundamental biological processes that drive aging.

CHAPTER 3

The Eternal Search for the Fountain of Youth

Youth is wasted on the young.
—*George Bernard Shaw,*
Irish-born author (1856–1950)

Everyone wants to go to heaven,
but nobody wants to die to get there.
—*Anonymous*

Nestled along Florida's sun-drenched east coast, Saint Augustine, a city not far from where I have lived for many years, feels like a place where history lingers in the air and time stands still. Founded in 1565, fifty-five years before the Pilgrims landed at Plymouth Rock and forty years before the English colonized Jamestown, it is the oldest permanent existing European settlement in all of North America. With its narrow cobblestone streets, centuries-old Spanish architecture, and moss-draped oak trees, it's a place where the past lives on. But this charming city with a small-town feel holds a legend far older than its walls—a tale that has intrigued and inspired for centuries: the story of the fountain of youth.

In 1515 the Spanish explorer Juan Ponce de León sailed from Spain to the New World, driven by the promise of new lands and untold riches. But according to legend, after hearing stories from Taino Indians in the Caribbean, he sought something far more elusive: a magical spring whose waters could restore youth and grant eternal life. It was said to be hidden somewhere in the lush, uncharted lands of what we now call Florida, and in his quest, Ponce de León etched his name into the annals of mythology. While history suggests that his true motivations were more political, the legend took on a life of its own, entwining Ponce de León's name with the dream of eternal youth.

Today visitors to Saint Augustine can stroll through the tranquil Fountain of Youth Archaeological Park, where the myth comes alive amid the beauty of ancient trees and a bubbling spring. A beautiful building, the Spring House, includes the original spring that was actually recorded in a seventeenth-century Spanish land grant. Tourists sip from the waters, if only for the thrill of imagining that they've tapped into the secret to everlasting youth.

Many historians believe that Ponce de León never searched for the fountain of youth, but the legend continues to this day. Although we don't know of a single spring that can reverse time, the desire behind the myth has never left us. The concept of a fountain of youth speaks to something timeless: the deep-rooted human longing to stay young and defy aging; to hold on to life's vitality just a little longer.

The Search for Youthful Longevity in Ancient Times

As a physician fascinated by the history of medicine in general, and longevity in particular, I'm continually amazed by humanity's timeless quest for youth and vitality. Let me take you through this remarkable journey that has shaped my own perspective on longevity.

When I study the ancient Egyptians, I'm struck by their sophisticated understanding of preservation and vitality. These weren't just primitive practitioners; they were pioneering medical innovators of their time. Their meticulous mummification processes, dating back to around 2600 BC, went beyond mere burial rituals; they symbolized humanity's earliest systematic attempt to preserve biological integrity indefinitely. What particularly intrigues me is their advanced pharmacological knowledge. For example, the Egyptians developed complex botanical formulations—combining potent natural oils, medicinal herbs, and therapeutic compounds such as honey and aloe—creating what we might consider the world's first anti-aging protocols.

The ancient Greeks and Romans then elevated this pursuit to new heights, developing what I see as the foundations of modern integrative medicine. I'm particularly inspired by the holistic approach of Hippocrates (460 –377 BC) , the Greek physician widely regarded today as the father of medicine. His recognition of hydrotherapy's therapeutic potential and emphasis on physical activity and dietary discipline mirror many principles we still apply in contemporary regenerative medicine. The Romans' sophisticated public baths weren't just social centers—they were comprehensive wellness facilities. When I think about the influential Greek physician and writer Galen (AD 129–216) and his contributions to surgical techniques and pharmacology, I see the beginnings of evidence-based interventional approaches to maintaining physical vigor.

The medieval period (from about AD 500 to 1500), often dismissed as an era of superstition, actually witnessed remarkable experimentation in longevity research. The alchemists, despite their mystical reputation, were essentially early biochemists. Their methodical search for the elixir of life parallels our current pursuit of cellular regeneration therapies. Their work went far beyond attempting to transform lead into gold using a mythical substance called the "philosopher's stone"—they were attempting to understand and manipulate the fundamental processes of biological aging, much as we do today with molecular and cellular interventions.

The Renaissance period, spanning the fourteenth through seventeenth centuries, particularly resonates with me as a modern practitioner. Leonardo da Vinci's precise anatomical studies laid the groundwork for our understanding of human biology. His belief that comprehending the body's mechanics could lead to methods of mitigating aging aligns perfectly with our current approach to regenerative medicine. Even Ponce de León's seemingly fantastical quest for the fountain of youth reflects a fundamental truth I've observed in my practice: nature often holds the keys to biological regeneration. I think that the Spanish explorer, just like you and me, was also in search of youthfulness more than just longevity.

What fascinates me most about this historical journey is how it mirrors our current endeavors in regenerative medicine. Each era contributed vital pieces to our understanding: the Egyptians' expertise in preservation techniques, the Greco-Roman emphasis on holistic wellness, the alchemists' pursuit of cellular transformation, and the Renaissance's integration of systematic observation with bold exploration.

As I try to apply cutting-edge regenerative and anti-aging therapies in my everyday practice, I'm deeply aware that it is all building upon this rich historical foundation. The same fundamental questions that intrigued ancient healers—how to maintain vitality, prevent decline, and optimize human potential—continue to guide our modern research and clinical innovations. The key difference is that we now have the scientific tools and understanding to transform these age-old aspirations into clinical realities.

This historical perspective reminds me constantly that while our methods have evolved dramatically, our fundamental mission remains unchanged: to help humans achieve optimal health and longevity. It's truly humbling to me to be part of this continuing journey that began with the ancient Egyptians and extends into our modern era of precision regenerative medicine.

The Search Continues in Modern Times

In the modern era, the hunger for youth and longevity has not changed, it has merely become more sophisticated and science-driven, with a greater focus on understanding and manipulating the fundamental biological processes that promote aging. This is good, I believe, as long as we don't lose sight of the fact that we should continue to advance the science of longevity for the sake of humanity as a whole, and not just for the few fortunate ones who can afford it. From genetics and regenerative medicine, to the integration of artificial intelligence in healthcare, today's researchers are on the brink of significant breakthroughs in human longevity. Here let us enter the world of the famous and ultra-wealthy looking for the same fountain of youth in our times using the latest technologies currently available. *Imagine being able to buy almost anything in the world, except time.* That's the fascinating paradox facing today's ultra-wealthy, who are now devoting their considerable resources to help develop innovative technologies to extend healthspan and lifespan as much as possible.

Enter our modern-day explorers—not wearing pith helmets and carrying maps but armed with billions of dollars and cutting-edge technology. Take Jeff Bezos, for instance. Here's a man who transformed how we shop, read, and live our daily lives through Amazon, and now he's set his sights on perhaps the most ambitious delivery of all: extending human life. When you think about it, it's rather poetic—the same person who made same-day shipping possible is now investing in making our own biological clocks run longer and better.

Bezos has poured significant resources into the biotechnology company Altos Labs, founded in 2022, where some of the world's brightest minds are not just studying aging but are looking at how to rewind it at a cellular level. Imagine your cells as tiny clocks that have been ticking away since birth—these scientists are trying to figure out if we can turn those hands back, even just a little bit. It's like trying to edit a document that's been writing itself for decades.

What makes this story particularly interesting is how personal it is. These billionaires aren't just throwing money at abstract concepts from their ivory towers. Bezos, for instance, has transformed his own lifestyle, becoming a fitness enthusiast in his late fifties. It's a reminder that beneath the billions and the cutting-edge science, there's something deeply human at play: the desire to live longer, healthier lives.

And Bezos isn't alone in this high-stakes scientific adventure. Peter Thiel, known for seeing the future before others do (he was, after all, an early Facebook investor), has joined forces with Bezos to back Unity Biotechnology, a company headquartered in San Francisco. Researchers there are tackling something called *senescent cells*. Think of them as the grumpy old cells in our body that refuse to call it a day gracefully and instead cause mischief in the form of arthritis and eye problems. Unity's mission is both bold and precise: it wants to find ways to either retire these troublemakers or induce them to behave.

Larry Ellison, cofounder of the computer technology company Oracle, has his own stake in this race against time. He's investing heavily in companies such as Life Biosciences and Human Longevity, the latter of which was launched by the celebrated biochemist-geneticist Craig Venter, a primary force behind the landmark effort to decipher all the approximately twenty thousand genes in human DNA. Meanwhile, entrepreneur Sam Altman—yes, the same person making waves with OpenAI and ChatGPT these days—has made an intriguing move by investing $180 million in Retro Biosciences. The California-based company, which states its mission to one day extend human life by a decade, is doing remarkable work with *T lymphocytes*, the special forces of our immune system. Imagine being able to modify these cellular warriors, better known as T cells, by genetically engineering them to potentially slow down or reverse aging and to fight off cancer and infections. And with Altman's expertise in AI, there's potential for machine learning to discover new combinations of treatments we humans might never have thought of.

The story gets even more interesting with the involvement of Meta CEO Mark Zuckerberg and his wife, Priscilla Chan. Along with Google's Sergey Brin, they established the Breakthrough Prize—think of it as the Academy Awards for scientists working on extending human life. It's their way of saying, "Hey, if you're brilliant and working on helping us live longer, healthier lives, we want to support you."

What's particularly fascinating is how this modern quest for longevity brings together different worlds. You have the raw computing power of artificial intelligence, the precision of genetic engineering, the persistence of traditional medical research, and the virtually unlimited resources of tech billionaires—all focused on solving one of humanity's oldest desires: more time.

One pivotal concept within the scientific community, shaping this seismic push toward eternal life, is this revolutionary shift in the paradigm of aging itself. What was once accepted as an inevitable decline is now being recognized and challenged as a potentially modifiable biological process. Through my extensive work in regenerative and longevity medicine, I've observed how this fundamental shift in perspective is transforming our approach to longevity and health optimization. We will discuss this more in chapter 6.

Imagine a world where we don't just live longer, but stay healthy, active, and sharp well into our later years. Where diseases that we now accept as inevitable parts of aging become as treatable as the common cold. That's the vision these modern pioneers are striving to achieve.

This isn't just about helping the ultra-wealthy live longer. The breakthroughs being pursued today could eventually transform how all of us age. The way I look at it is that, in the end, it's really a story of human ambition, hope, and possibility. While their bank accounts might be extraordinary, these billionaires share this same fundamental human desire you and I have—the wish to have more time with loved ones, more years to pursue dreams, more moments to experience the joy of being alive. As billionaires dive into the world of longevity science, they are reshaping the future of how we understand aging, offering a glimpse of what might be possible in the years to come—not just for the ultra-wealthy, but for humanity as a whole.

So, Can Money *Really* Buy Health and Longevity?

It is widely reported that, after his polio diagnosis in 1921 at the age of thirty-nine, future US president Franklin D. Roosevelt pursued numerous holistic, alternative treatments, both in the United States and abroad, to manage his paralysis and strive for mobility. Throughout his twelve years as the thirty-second commander in chief, FDR spent whatever time he could in Warm Springs, Georgia, at the quaint six-room retreat he'd built there dubbed the Little White House—and not just to seek a respite from the pressures of the Oval Office. In 1924 he'd visited a resort in town after having heard about a young man with polio who'd claimed that immersing himself in its mountain water pools had prompted his recovery. The very first time Roosevelt went swimming, he experienced some improvement. In the end, though, he never regained full mobility in his legs. FDR was said to have traveled to Europe in search of experimental treatments popular at the time. It was not uncommon—then or now—for the wealthy and powerful to seek alternative therapies, and his journeys reflect the lengths that high-profile figures will go to pursue advanced but unconventional medical treatments, hoping for improvements in health and longevity.

Across Europe, luxury wellness clinics and resorts are gaining a reputation for offering some of the world's most exclusive and advanced regenerative and longevity treatments, attracting billionaires and Hollywood celebrities alike. These clinics now provide the latest programs that tap into the body's regenerative capabilities, promoting healing and revitalization at a cellular level. Such therapies, once considered experimental, have become increasingly refined and accessible to those who seek them, positioning Europe as a global hub for those in pursuit of longevity and vitality.

Nestled in scenic locations like the Swiss Alps or secluded parts of Austria and Germany, these clinics are known for both discretion and high-end luxury, where guests come not only for privacy but also for access to experimental treatments unavailable or heavily regulated in the United States. Although the exact therapies offered are often shrouded in confidentiality, my research suggests that such clinics provide services ranging from placental stem cell, young blood transfusions, exosome infusions, and cellular rejuvenation therapies to anti-aging protocols targeting inflammation and cellular repair. Many of these regenerative treatments are believed to enhance energy, reverse diseases, improve skin elasticity, and extend lifespan.

The costs of such treatments are exorbitant, often ranging from tens of thousands of dollars to hundreds of thousands of dollars for a single program. People stay in opulent surroundings, complete with private villas, world-class spa facilities, and personal chefs catering to highly specific dietary needs. These clinics are designed to serve every detail of their clients' health and comfort, offering customized wellness programs that include personalized nutrition, fitness regimes, and regenerative therapies. For those who can afford it, the promise of turning back the biological clock comes wrapped in the utmost luxury and privacy.

While the efficacy and safety of some of these regenerative treatments remain a subject of debate, the demand continues to grow. The ultra-wealthy are willing to take their chances with experimental therapies that could potentially offer a fountain of youth. The allure of a longer, more vibrant life—coupled with the exclusivity of these clinics—makes these European wellness sanctuaries the ideal destination for those seeking the ultimate in health and luxury, all away from the prying eyes of the public.

From Eons to Now

As we discussed, what sets today's search for youthfulness and longevity apart from past efforts is its grounding in robust science and the convergence of multiple fields of research. By unraveling the complexities of aging through genomics (branch of molecular biology dealing with study of entire genes), cellular biology, and advanced technologies, today's researchers are on the cusp of significant breakthroughs that could transform human longevity in ways previously unimaginable. For the first time, the idea of reversing or significantly slowing aging no longer belongs in the realm of myth but is becoming a scientific reality.

The twentieth century brought what I consider a paradigm shift with the dawn of molecular biology, as well as the discovery of deoxyribonucleic acid, or DNA—the long molecule in every cell that contains genes, which in turn carry biological instructions necessary for life—and genomics. As a practitioner, I'm now able to evaluate and influence the very genetic pathways that control aging: telomere dynamics, cellular senescence mechanisms, and mitochondrial function. The advent of stem cell technology has been particularly revolutionary in my practice, offering unprecedented potential for tissue regeneration and cellular rejuvenation. We will discuss these in detail in chapters that follow.

What excites me most is how artificial intelligence and advanced analytics are transforming our clinical approach. In my practice, I can now utilize AI-driven algorithms to optimize personalized treatment protocols for my patients and to assess their biological aging with remarkable precision. This technological integration allows us to move beyond symptomatic treatment to address aging's root causes at the molecular level. The potential of CRISPR gene-editing technology to modify DNA in living organisms particularly fascinates me—it represents a quantum leap in our ability to potentially correct age-related genetic modifications.

Looking back over the past five decades of anti-aging medicine, it is fascinating to see the evolution from basic interventions such as traditional surgical facelifts and vitamin supplementation to sophisticated hormone replacement protocols, laser rejuvenation procedures, and targeted stem cell therapies. While our methods have become more sophisticated, the fundamental goal remains unchanged: optimizing human health and longevity.

In my practice, I've seen these advanced therapies offer new hope to patients struggling with age-related decline, chronic conditions, and degenerative diseases. The convergence of ancient wisdom with cutting-edge science has brought us to an unprecedented moment in medical history. For the first time, we're not just dreaming about reversing biological aging—we're developing concrete strategies to achieve it.

Now, we arrive at the VitalLife program, which embodies the essence of everything I have learned over four decades of medical practice about optimizing human health, wellness, and vitality. In the next chapter, let us delve into this transformative program.

CHAPTER 4

The VitalLife Program: An Overview

> There comes a point where we need to stop just pulling people out of the river. We need to go upstream and find out why they are falling in.
> —*Bishop Desmond Tutu, South African bishop and human rights activist (1931–2021)*

> The two most important days in your life are the day you are born and the day you find out why.
> —*Mark Twain, celebrated American writer and humorist (1835–1910)*

At fifty-six, Tom seemed to have it all. He'd climbed the corporate ladder to become a senior executive at a Fortune 100 company, built a loving family with his wife and two children, and checked all the boxes of conventional success. Yet when he looked in the mirror each morning, something felt missing: that spark, that fire that once defined him. He had settled into the belief that his best days were behind him. It wasn't as though it had happened overnight, but over the years, he had slowly felt age creeping in—stealing his energy, his drive, and even the quiet confidence he once took for granted. He remembered a time when he could wake up, hit the ground running, and face the world without hesitation. His strength was undeniable, his mind sharp, and the idea of slowing down was as foreign to him as the thought of getting old.

But now, the feeling of "I'm getting older" was harder to ignore for Tom. His mornings started slower, his body no longer responding with the ease it once did. Small aches that he used to shrug off became daily companions. Even his once unshakeable self-assurance seemed to have dulled, replaced by a resignation that maybe this was just how life goes. Like so many, he began to believe that perhaps aging truly meant getting weaker, less capable, and somehow . . . *less alive*.

Yet there was still something inside him—a flicker of dissatisfaction, a question that wouldn't go away. What if this wasn't the only way forward? What if getting older didn't have to mean accepting decline? Tom began to wonder: Maybe, just maybe, aging could be a time to evolve into an even stronger, wiser, and more vibrant man than he had ever been. He imagined a life where each day felt as full of possibility as the days of his youth. The thought stayed with him, small at first, but growing stronger with time. What if fifty-six wasn't the beginning of the end but rather the start of a new chapter—one in which he felt more alive than ever before?

One day while waiting in the airline's club lounge for his flight at New York's Kennedy International Airport, Tom read a magazine article about how, as our youthfulness starts diminishing, so many people stop enjoying life, and then, slowly, stop even trying. Before they realize it, they have resigned themselves to the situation, and then life itself fades away.

Something clicked. That ember burst into flame. What if aging wasn't a slow surrender to decline, he pondered, but a gateway—a threshold—to a life more luminous, a chapter bursting with vitality and richness yet to be discovered? He decided to act. This realization led Tom to my office to regain what seemed like a lost part of his life. He came to my office seeking not just medical treatment but also a rekindling of his spirit. After a thorough medical evaluation that included a full diagnostic workup, he was started on a comprehensive and personalized VitalLife program.

After just four weeks on this data-driven, science-backed, comprehensive, and personalized program tailored to his biology, Tom's transformation was remarkable. He started feeling better physically, more energetic. Perhaps more importantly, he felt hopeful, passionate, and joyous about life again.

Tom's story isn't unique. Now, imagine yourself in this story. What if the energy of your youth wasn't just a memory? *What if your best days weren't behind you, but ahead?* What if each morning could bring a sense of renewed possibility, with a body and mind ready to embrace life's adventures? This program can become your road map to those transformations, too. Like Tom, you too can write a new chapter—one where age becomes not a limitation, but a launching pad to your most vibrant self. Here is the defining truth that forms the very essence of the VitalLife program: you do have the power to reverse biological age and modify your genetic blueprint, heralding a future where longevity and vitality intertwine.

A Proven Program of Twenty Years

We are all familiar with this: temporary fixes for fatigue, stress, and dwindling vitality —such as caffeine, alcohol, medications, or stimulants —may provide fleeting relief, but they merely mask the underlying issue of cellular dysfunction. Through decades of clinical research and experience, I've developed this VitalLife program: a comprehensive lifestyle system designed to *optimize health and longevity at the cellular level*. It's a science-backed program that harnesses cutting-edge advancements in regenerative medicine to rebuild the body from within. VitalLife provides a fundamentally different way to reclaim vitality and enduring health.

There are several other key factors that make this program so effective in optimizing healthspan and longevity. First, the success of this program lies in its precision. Built on sophisticated data analysis, biomarker optimization, and latest scientific advancements, every protocol is meticulously tailored to align with individual biology and personal goals.

> You do have the power to reverse biological age and modify your genetic blueprint, heralding a future where longevity and vitality intertwine.

Also, by merging advanced Western medical treatments with the timeless wisdom of Eastern healing, it offers a *comprehensive approach* that addresses the root causes of aging and disease. From cellular rejuvenation to hormonal optimization, metabolic regulation, and immune modulation, it goes far beyond what's available or possible with conventional medicine.

The Benefits of the VitalLife Program

You know what amazes me most after so many years of helping people with this program? It's not just the cutting-edge technology or the breakthrough treatments—it's the look in someone's eyes when they realize their best days aren't behind them. Here are some key benefits that patients of mine have reported over the years:

- **Renewed Energy and Recovery:** The VitalLife program supports healthy cellular and metabolic function to help you build healthy muscle tone, increase energy levels, and improve your overall physical and mental performance. So, whether lack of energy, strength, and stamina stems from an illness or is due to no apparent reason at all, people have experienced significant improvements in overall vitality.
- **Reduced Inflammation and Improved Immunity:** VitalLife helps strengthen your immune system and reduces inflammation throughout the body to stimulate

the body's natural healing mechanism, helps repair cellular damage, and promotes faster recovery.
- **Improved Muscle Mass and Strength:** The program helps prevent and treat dangerous *sarcopenia*, the age-related loss of muscle mass and quality. In addition, patients see an improvement in muscle strength, flexibility, performance, and stamina.
- **Improved Cognition and Mood:** VitalLife supports healthy brain function and mood. So, people experience reduced brain fog and a boost in cognition, memory, and happiness. In short, they feel like themselves again—or perhaps even better than before.
- **Better Sleep:** People on this program report significant improvement in sleep quality and duration. So, they wake up refreshed and ready to take on the world.
- **Enhanced Sexual Health:** VitalLife treats men's erectile dysfunction (ED), improving sexual performance, and, in both men and women, reignites the desire for intimacy.
- **Healthy Aging:** The program slows and even reverses biomarkers of aging and diseases, thus increasing your lifespan and, more importantly, your healthspan.

The Six Pillars of the VitalLife Program for Optimal Healthspan and Lifespan

Here are the six pillars to this cutting-edge, holistic approach to longevity that enhances both lifespan and healthspan. To achieve the best results for each person, for me it is of utmost importance to have a *personalized, data-driven, and comprehensive approach.* Through my years of clinical practice, I've *continuously refined many treatment modalities*, incorporating the latest technologies and clinical data to optimize outcomes.

One more important factor to keep in mind: In chapter 6, we will discuss in detail the processes of aging and age-related diseases, including heart disease, stroke, and Alzheimer's disease. While these are often labeled as diseases of aging, *they begin as early as adolescence*, influenced by genetics, lifestyle, and environmental factors. *In essence, they are diseases of childhood showing up in later years.* Therefore, initiating this program at a younger age, with a focus on prevention, requires significantly less effort than attempting to reverse a disease and regain energy and vitality later in life. Let me walk you through the six pillars of this program.

Pillar One: Personalized Assessment and Testing

The program starts with comprehensive biomarker testing, which I discuss at length in chapter 7. The cornerstone of this program is its emphasis on a personalized assessment and testing, conducted at the outset and then repeated at regular intervals to monitor progress in the right direction without any complications. Rather than relying on one-size-fits-all solutions, the program uses personalized biomarkers to assess aging markers, hormone levels, inflammation and immunity markers, and cognitive function.

Test for DNA methylation (a chemical process that adds a methyl group to DNA, which can regulate how our genes function) provides insights into biological age, while advanced screenings such as *Galleri cancer detection* proactively identify potential health risks. This precise, data-driven approach allows for the creation of a customized health plan, empowering individuals to take control of their aging process.

Pillar Two: Regenerative Medicine and Cellular Rejuvenation

At the heart of this program is its innovative use of regenerative medicine, which taps into the body's own repair mechanisms to combat aging at a cellular level. The science is also clear: *aging and its associated diseases can be addressed through appropriate regenerative treatments.* In chapters 8 and 9, we will explore various regenerative treatments, ranging from autologous stem cells derived from your own fat or bone marrow to placental stem cells, exosomes, and extracellular vesicles. The program harnesses many of these advanced therapies to rejuvenate tissues and organs.

Modern technologies like *senolytics* that remove toxic senescent cells, *therapeutic plasma exchange, ozone therapy, hyperbaric oxygen,* and *light therapy* support this regeneration. Although not a part of my program—I am closely watching the emerging and controversial field of *parabiosis* (transfusion of a young person's blood into an older person), used by several prominent figures and billionaires. It is discussed only as a *possible* option in the near future. These approaches, combined with the exploration of psychedelic therapies discussed in chapter 10 —including magic mushrooms and ketamine —provide a groundbreaking path to healing and anti-aging.

Pillar Three: Hormonal and Peptide Optimization

In chapter 11, you'll learn how an optimal hormonal balance is essential for maintaining energy, performance, and vitality as we age. This program offers personalized strategies to restore youthful levels of hormones such as testosterone, estrogen, progesterone, and growth hormone, as well as innovative peptides such as sermorelin, PT-141, and BPC-157. These therapies not only counteract the natural decline that occurs with aging but also enhance vitality, cognitive function, and sexual health. With a focus on precision and balance, the program ensures a symphony of hormones and peptides to support long-term health.

Pillar Four: Controlling the VitalLife Aging Triad of Mitochondrial Dysfunction, Metabolic Insulin Resistance, and Chronic Inflammation

The VitalLife Aging Triad, explored in detail in chapter 6, consists of three key cellular processes that closely interact with one another in a *cellular feedback loop* and are instrumental in causing aging and diseases of aging: (1) *mitochondrial dysfunction,* (2) *metabolic insulin resistance,* and (3) *systemic chronic low-grade inflammation.* I've discovered that targeting this root cause of aging offers the most promising approach to extending both healthspan and lifespan as well as reversing diseases. VitalLife incorporates various strategies to do just that.

Chapters 12 and 13 emphasize this particular focus on improving mitochondrial function and insulin sensitivity and reducing chronic inflammation. Special attention is given to the role of the gut microbiome, a key player in immune regulation and overall health. With dietary adjustments, supplements and medicines such as metformin and colchicine, the program fosters a robust immune system and youthful metabolic function.

Pillar Five: Personalized Compounded Medicines for Longevity and Health

As detailed in chapter 14, another key aspect of this program is its focus on *personalized medicine,* utilizing compounded medicines such as rapamycin, ketamine, and low-dose naltrexone to address specific health challenges and promote longevity. VitalLife also includes tailored peptides, intravenous (IV) infusions, and supplemental **NAD+**, a coenzyme that helps repair and energize cells, boosting cellular energy and promoting optimal function. Hormonal therapies are finely tuned for men and women, ensuring that the delicate balance of testosterone, estrogen, and progesterone is maintained for peak health and well-being.

Pillar Six: Transformative Lifestyle Modifications

As we will explore in chapter 5, studies on men and women who have made it to age one hundred or older (called centenarians) provide valuable insights into longevity. These include nurturing meaningful social relationships; engaging in regular brain training exercises; cultivating optimism, a sense of humor, and other positive personality traits; discovering your purpose; practicing gratitude; and embracing the act of giving.

Many of the lessons learned from centenarians are woven into this final pillar of the VitalLife Program. It focuses on lifestyle choices that influence longevity and vitality. Chapters 15 through 18 are devoted to this crucial aspect of the program.

In these chapters, we will discuss several key lifestyle factors: eating a whole-food, plant-based diet and avoiding processed and fried foods; environmental toxins; the importance of staying physically active; incorporating techniques to reduce chronic stress, such as meditation and yoga; and taking steps to ensure a sound sleep. My program strongly advocates first and foremost eliminating harmful habits, or what I call the *"unholy trinity"* of smoking, drinking alcohol, and eating processed foods that provide "tasty toxins"—all of which can undermine even the most effective youthfulness and anti-aging efforts. A focus on Blue Zone and whole-food, plant-based diets, and intermittent fasting promotes a healthy metabolism and reduces inflammation. Certain key proven longevity supplements and herbs further support disease-modifying and anti-aging efforts. The program also emphasizes strength training to prevent a serious condition called sarcopenia that results in muscle loss, and mindfulness practices like meditation and yoga to enhance mental resilience and emotional well-being.

By creating an integrated and personalized plan for each individual by *combining many of these powerful elements* as required based on each person's health history and objective medical data, you get an unparalleled approach to attaining peak health outcomes.

The Medical Conditions Improved

Through years of treating patients with this program, I've observed and measured its transformative effects, often hearing directly from patients about the remarkable improvements they've experienced in their medical conditions, overall health, and longevity.

- **Longevity and Senescence:** People feel tired, have experience memory issues and declining stamina as they age. Like many scientists around the world, I too believe that the effects and diseases of aging are biological processes that can be slowed or even reversed with appropriate regenerative and other treatments.
- **Chronic Diseases**—Regenerative medicine helps regulate cell function in the body. People report significant improvements in vitality and health with VitalLife when suffering from diseases of the heart, brain, lungs, immunity, or metabolism. Whether your concerns are due to autoimmune diseases, metabolic conditions such as diabetes and obesity, long COVID, or degenerative diseases of aging such as heart disease, stroke, and Alzheimer's, various individualized treatment protocols in this program can help.
- **Brain Health:** Research around the globe shows various regenerative therapies and psychedelics can help brain health and wellness, traumatic brain injuries, and neurodegenerative diseases such as Alzheimer's, Parkinson's disease, and dementia.
- **Immunity and Inflammation Diseases:** Using regenerative therapies, scientists, physicians, and patients from around the globe have reported improvements in immune function in diseases such as rheumatoid arthritis, lupus, celiac disease, Crohn's disease, diabetes, and even long COVID syndrome.
- **Mental Illnesses:** With a comprehensive psychedelic ketamine program along with other regenerative protocols, people have seen tremendous improvements in their mental wellness. They feel decreases in anxiety, depression,

post-traumatic stress disorder (PTSD), chronic pain, and insomnia.
- **Athletic Performance:** I have more than twenty years of experience healing injuries and improving performance in professional athletes from the NFL and NHL; I've worked with athletes from the soccer, tennis, and other sports. As we will discuss in detail in the following chapters, regenerative therapies help increase performance and avoid dangerous surgeries for sports injuries.

In order to ensure optimal results and avoid any side effects, I meticulously track, at regular intervals, many biomarker and biological age tests. This allows for continuously monitoring progress and adjusting protocols based on objective data and each patient's clinical response.

Understanding the benefits of the VitalLife program is an important first step, but the real power lies in grasping the *how* and *why* behind this approach. When you understand the science and the strategies, you'll feel truly empowered to implement these principles in your own life. In the next chapter, we'll dive into the root causes of aging and disease—how they manifest and why addressing these underlying factors is significantly more effective than merely treating symptoms or chasing test results. By clearly understanding the root cause, you'll gain better insight into what makes the VitalLife program so effective.

PART 2

UNDERSTANDING THE SCIENCE OF AGING

CHAPTER 5

Unraveling the Mysteries of Aging: The Science of Why We Age

Aging is the greatest of all puzzles; to solve it is to unlock the deepest secrets of life.
—Friedrich Nietzsche, German philosopher (1844–1900)

The longer I live, the more I observe that the key to everything rests in the science of the body.
—Leonardo da Vinci, Italian polymath (1452–1519)

We know that aging is a process that affects every part of our body, yet few of us truly understand *why* and *how* it happens. Let me share something interesting: The real story of aging unfolds deep within our cells. You might notice it as wrinkles in the mirror or feeling tired more often. Perhaps you're concerned about heart health or other age-related conditions. But what I want you to understand is that these visible signs are just the tip of the iceberg.

Advances in science, research, and technology have opened the door to a much deeper understanding of how our bodies function, not only when we're battling illnesses but also as we age. We now know that aging isn't simply a matter of the years ticking by; it's driven by a series of internal and external factors that affect our cells and tissues at the most fundamental levels. Within the body, cellular processes—compounded by external toxins from our environment—lead to increased inflammation, oxidative stress, and even damage to our DNA. These factors accelerate the aging process, causing premature wear and tear on our cells.

You might be surprised to learn that *the cellular changes we associate with getting older can begin as early as your twenties.* Yes, even while you're reveling in the vitality of youth, your cells are quietly undergoing changes that will shape your future health. By the time symptoms appear, the underlying disease processes may have been developing in your body for years, even decades. But this knowledge is empowering, for the earlier we recognize these changes and address them, the better the outcome.

In this chapter, *we'll explore how multiple biological factors interact with one another in contributing to the aging process.* I've come to see the human body as nature's most sophisticated symphony—far more complex than any of Beethoven's masterpieces. Think of the immune system as the string section, the endocrine system as the brass, while the nervous system keeps time like percussion, and the cardiovascular system flows like woodwinds.

What fascinates me most is how a slight discord in one system—like an out-of-tune immune response—creates ripples of disharmony throughout our entire biological orchestra. I've observed how chronic inflammation acts like a gradually detuning instrument, subtly altering the body's symphony until it loses its coherence. Just as a conductor doesn't focus solely on a single musician but directs the entire orchestra, we must approach healing with this same holistic vision. Through proper interventions, we can restore the magnificent coherence that characterizes optimal health—bringing back the symphony written in our genes and conducted by our cellular processes.

> Aging is not something that just happens to us. It is not a one-way street. By understanding the underlying science of aging, we can influence the way we age by making informed choices.

As researchers continue to unlock the secrets of aging, one thing is clear: aging is not simply something that happens to us. We can influence the way we age by making informed choices about our lifestyle, diet, and personalized health strategies. Understanding the science of aging gives us the power to take control of our health in ways that weren't possible before. The body's systems are intricate, but once we know how to manage things like inflammation and support mitochondrial health, we can begin to slow the aging process and improve our quality of life.

You might be wondering, *Can I really influence how I age?* Based on my clinical experience, *the answer is a resounding YES.* Every day in my practice, I help patients take control of their aging process. Whether they're in their thirties looking to prevent age-related changes, or in their sixties seeking to revitalize their health, the principles remain the same. It's about understanding and working with your body's natural processes.

In the chapters that follow, you'll learn exactly how this program targets these cellular mechanisms that cause aging and diseases to help you maintain vitality and health. I've seen countless patients achieve remarkable results by applying these principles, and I'm confident you can, too. All it takes is understanding how your body works and giving it what it needs to thrive.

Lessons from Centenarians: Unlocking the Secrets to a Long, Healthy Life

Centenarians—those remarkable individuals who have lived for a century or more—grant us an extraordinary glimpse into the secrets of a long and fulfilling life. Their experiences and habits provide invaluable lessons, guiding us to pave our own journey toward longevity. Through my extensive study of these remarkable lives, I have woven countless insights into my VitalLife program, enabling my patients to embark on their own empowering health journeys.

Across the globe, researchers have dedicated decades to studying these extraordinary individuals to uncover the factors that contribute to their remarkable health and vitality. Major studies, including the Blue Zones Project, a community-wide initiative, and the Okinawa Centenarian Study from the Okinawa Research Center for Longevity Science, in Japan, have revealed powerful lessons about how to live longer, healthier lives.

The Blue Zones Project, started in 2004, identified five regions of the world with unusually high concentrations of centenarians: (1) Okinawa, Japan, (2) Sardinia, Italy, (3) Nicoya, Costa Rica, (4) Ikaria, Greece, and (5) Loma Linda, California. These studies showed that longevity is not tied to genetics alone—in fact, environmental, lifestyle, and social factors play an even larger role. The centenarians in these regions shared common traits, including strong social connections, regular physical activity, plant-based diets, and an enduring sense of purpose, known in Okinawa as *ikigai*.

Similarly, the Okinawa Centenarian Study, one of the most comprehensive investigations into healthy aging, has followed more than nine hundred centenarians in Okinawa since the 1970s. The findings consistently highlight the importance of a calorie-conscious, nutrient-dense diet rich in vegetables, whole grains, and lean proteins, particularly tofu and moderate amounts of fish. These individuals also emphasize community, with many centenarians there actively participating in social groups called *moai*, which provide emotional support and foster resilience.

From these studies, several actionable lessons emerge for anyone striving to live a longer and healthier life and these are helpful in designing one's own optimal healthspan plan, such as VitalLife:

- **Nurture Meaningful Relationships**: Social isolation has been shown to have severe health consequences.

Foster strong bonds with family, friends, and your community to improve emotional resilience and physical health.
- **Stay Active, Naturally**: Rather than structured workouts, centenarians integrate movement into their daily lives through gardening, walking, or manual work. Regular, moderate activity helps maintain muscle strength, cardiovascular health, and mobility.
- **Adopt a Plant-Based Diet:** Most centenarians consume a diet rich in fruits, vegetables, beans, and whole grains, with limited red meat and processed foods. Small portions and mindful eating are common themes.
- **Find Your Purpose:** Having a clear reason to wake up each morning—whether it's family, work, or hobbies—provides motivation and reduces stress. This sense of purpose contributes significantly to mental well-being.
- **Reduce Stress**: Centenarians often practice daily rituals that lower stress, such as prayer, meditation, or simply enjoying time with loved ones. Stress management is critical for reducing inflammation and protecting overall health.
- **Sleep Well:** A consistent sleep routine ensures physical and cognitive recovery, which are essential for longevity.
- **Maintain a Positive Mindset**: Centenarians are often easygoing, quick to laugh, and rarely hold on to anger or grudges. This lighthearted approach to life, coupled with gratitude and resilience, fosters emotional well-being and reduces stress.
- **Keep Your Brain Active**: Centenarians prioritize mental stimulation through lifelong learning, puzzles, reading, and social interactions. Keeping the brain active helps maintain cognitive function and reduces the risk of dementia.
- **Practice Giving and Charity**: Many centenarians find fulfillment in helping others, whether through

volunteering, acts of kindness, or giving to their communities. This generosity strengthens social bonds and provides a sense of purpose and connection.

These lessons remind us that longevity isn't about perfection; it's about balance. By embracing these principles, we can move closer to a life that's not only longer but also rich in health, purpose, and joy.

Hallmarks of Aging

The scientific understanding of aging has undergone a revolutionary transformation in recent years. In 2013 a groundbreaking framework emerged from European scientists that fundamentally changed our approach to aging medicine: the Hallmarks of Aging. This sophisticated model outlined the biological mechanisms underlying everything from visible aging to age-related diseases.

What makes this framework particularly fascinating is its comprehensive approach to understanding aging's molecular and cellular foundations. In my clinical practice, I've seen how targeting these specific hallmarks can significantly slow down the biological aging processes.

The original nine hallmarks identified in 2013 have since been expanded to twelve, reflecting our deepening understanding of aging's complexity. Through careful clinical observation and advancing research, these hallmarks have proven to be fundamental targets for age management interventions.

Twelve Hallmarks That Drive Biological Aging

1. **Genomic Instability**: DNA replication errors and chromosomal defects compromise your genetic integrity, fundamentally affecting cellular health.

2. **Telomere Attrition**: These protective chromosomal structures gradually shorten, acting as a biological clock for cellular aging.
3. **Epigenetic Alterations**: Epigenetics is studying how environment effects your gene expression. Changes in DNA methylation patterns disrupt normal gene activity, affecting how your cells express genetic information.
4. **Proteostasis Dysfunction**: Proteostasis is the regulation of proteins within a cell. Disrupting that balance can impair essential cellular functions and bring about disease.
5. **Disabled Autophagy**: A progressive decline in your body's crucial ability to recycle damaged cellular components.
6. **Deregulated Nutrient Sensing**: Impairment of the cellular mechanisms for detecting and responding to beneficial nutrients such as glucose, amino acids, and fatty acids.
7. **Mitochondrial Dysfunction**: The cellular energy powerhouses called *mitochondria* deteriorate, compromising energy production and cellular vitality.
8. **Cellular Senescence**: An accumulation of nondividing but metabolically active cells that release harmful compounds, damaging surrounding tissues.
9. **Stem Cell Exhaustion:** A depletion of regenerative stem cell populations reduces the body's capacity for tissue repair.
10. **Altered Intercellular Communication**: A breakdown in cellular signaling leads to systemic dysfunction and inflammatory cascades.
11. **Systemic Chronic Inflammation**: Persistent low-grade inflammation throughout your body progressively damages tissues and accelerates aging.
12. **Dysbiosis**: Age-related changes in gut microbiome (bacteria, viruses, and fungi) composition influences systemic health and longevity.

What's particularly compelling about these hallmarks is their *intricate interconnectedness*. These pathways don't operate in isolation but instead form a complex network that collectively determines your aging trajectory. In my clinical experience, addressing multiple hallmarks simultaneously often yields the most significant results in biological age reduction.

Understanding these hallmarks has revolutionized our approach to longevity medicine. This isn't just theoretical science—it's the foundation for practical interventions that can meaningfully impact your biological aging process. Through careful monitoring and targeted interventions, we can now influence these fundamental aging processes.

Exploring the Main Theories of Aging: Unlocking the Mysteries of Longevity

Over the years, scientists have delved into the mysteries of aging, proposing fascinating theories to explain why we age. From senescent cells and chronic inflammation to epigenetic influences, the process of aging is a complex puzzle with many interconnected pieces. By exploring these widely accepted theories, we can begin to uncover the intricate mechanisms at work and gain a deeper understanding of this natural yet profoundly curious journey.

Why delve into what may seem like the mundane science of aging? Because by understanding these theories, we gain a deeper appreciation for the intricate mechanisms at work, uncovering ways to reverse our biological age and enhance both healthspan and longevity. By exploring this science, we empower ourselves with the knowledge to make informed and strategic decisions about when and how to apply various treatments—such as regenerative therapies, lifestyle adjustments, and innovative technologies—unlocking their full potential for optimal health, vitality, and longevity.

Let us now explore some of the most widely accepted and intriguing theories that illuminate this process of aging.

Senescent Cells in Aging Process

One of science's most compelling discoveries in past decades involves the pivotal role of senescent cells—commonly known as "zombie cells"—in the aging process. These cells have become central to work in anti-aging and regenerative medicine, fundamentally shaping our understanding of cellular aging mechanisms.

When a cell can no longer function properly, or divide, or repair itself, it is said to have entered this *senescent state*. While this process, first described in 1961, begins as a stable growth arrest triggered by various internal and external factors, its accumulating effects set off a cascade of age-related dysfunction. Multiple factors lead to senescence, such as chronic inflammation, mitochondrial dysfunction, and stem cell exhaustion, and there is an intimate link between this and other hallmarks of aging. Scientists have uncovered how cellular senescence manifests as cells experience stress and damage throughout their life cycles.

What I find particularly fascinating is the *complex interplay between senescent cells and immune function*. In younger people, the immune system efficiently eliminates these dysfunctional cells. However, with age, this crucial clearance mechanism becomes compromised, leading to zombie cells accumulating in the body's tissues.

The issue with senescent cells is that they don't just sit quietly in the body; *they release harmful chemicals,* inflammatory molecules called cytokines, toxic proteins, and other damaging cellular factors *into their surroundings*. This process, known as the *senescence-associated secretory phenotype* (*SASP*), generates persistent low-grade systemic inflammation (often called *inflammaging*) that damages nearby healthy cells and tissues. SASP is linked to many of the diseases associated with aging.

Zombie cells impair cellular function in every area of the body. In vascular tissues, they contribute to atherosclerotic plaque formation, increasing cardiovascular risk. In joint spaces, they degrade cartilage through cellular mediators, leading to osteoarthritis. In the liver and the pancreas, they disrupt insulin-signaling pathways and glucose homeostasis, potentially precipitating diabetes and *metabolic syndrome* (a cluster of conditions that increase the risk of developing chronic diseases such as heart disease and stroke). Perhaps most concerning is their contribution to cognitive decline and neurodegeneration.

Because senescent cells are implicated in so many age-related conditions, they've become a major target in anti-aging research. Scientists are exploring *senolytic drugs* that specifically target and remove senescent cells from the body. Early studies in animals have shown promising results.

Researchers are also investigating ways to enhance the immune system's ability to naturally clear senescent cells or to prevent cells from becoming senescent in the first place. The hope is that by homing in on these zombie cells, we can not only slow the aging process but also reduce the risk of many age-related diseases and improve the quality of life as we age.

VitalLife incorporates cutting-edge senolytic therapies that don't merely slow the aging process but also can actively reverse many age-related cellular changes, as evidenced by clinical observations and biomarker tests. From my own perspective, the benefits to patients are particularly impressive when we initiate treatment during earlier stages of cellular dysfunction.

What I want you to understand is that addressing cellular senescence isn't just about extending lifespan—it's about optimizing your healthspan. The science of senescent cells has revolutionized our approach to aging, offering unprecedented opportunities to maintain cellular vitality throughout life.

The Immune Cell Theory of Aging

The immune cell theory of aging reveals profound insights into biological decline, emphasizing how the immune system's gradual deterioration drives aging and age-related diseases. *Immunosenescence*, the process that weakens both *innate immunity* (what you are born with) and *adaptive immunity* (what immune cells learn and how they adapt as we grow), leads to reduced immune cell production, diminished cell effectiveness, and the accumulation of senescent immune cells. These changes increase a person's vulnerability to infections, cancers, and chronic diseases. Reversing these immune shifts offers hope for slowing aging and enhancing longevity.

In youth, the immune system efficiently fights pathogens, clears damaged cells, and supports tissue repair. However, with age, the thymus—a tiny, butterfly-shaped organ located just behind your breastbone, and the body's primary factory for turning out effective T cells—shrinks, limiting production. This decline, known as *thymic involution*, weakens the immune response, leaving older adults more susceptible to infections and cancers and slower to heal from wounds and other injuries. T cells lose their ability to coordinate the immune system's defense forces, further compromising immunity.

The immune cell theory of aging not only highlights immune decline but also underscores potential intervention strategies. Breaking the cycle of immunosenescence and inflammation requires targeting both processes. Emerging therapies to rejuvenate immune cells may slow aging and extend healthspan, offering promising avenues for clinical innovation.

Systemic Chronic Inflammation (SCI): A Key Factor in Aging

I believe that chronic, low-grade inflammation, or *inflammaging*, is one of the most critical factors driving biological aging and diseases of aging. While insulin resistance, mitochondrial dysfunction, and senescent cells play significant roles, I've observed through my clinical practice, my family's health struggles, and even my own health challenges that managing this silent, body-wide inflammation is essential for any successful vitality or longevity program, or for disease reversal.

Inflammaging is the body's natural inflammatory response gone awry. In acute cases, such as healing a cut or fighting an infection, inflammation is protective. But let it persist for years, even at a low level, and it becomes harmful, damaging tissues and organs, accelerating aging, and increasing the risk of chronic diseases such as cardiovascular disease, type 2 diabetes, Alzheimer's, and even certain forms of cancer.

So, what fuels this chronic inflammation? Contributors include a declining immune system, metabolic dysfunction, environmental toxins, and accumulation of senescent cells. Over time, the immune system weakens, becoming less effective at managing threats. This leads to a perpetual cycle of low-grade activation, cellular damage, and further immune weakening—an endless loop that accelerates aging and disease progression.

> Whole-body chronic inflammation, a slow-simmering fire, is the *"common denominator"* behind aging and diseases of aging, including cardiovascular disease, stroke, Alzheimer's, diabetes, arthritis, and even cancer.

One of the most fascinating connections I've seen is between the gut microbiome and systemic inflammation. Your gut, home to trillions of microorganisms, is a master regulator of immune responses. When the gut microbiome falls into imbalance (dysbiosis), it disrupts the intestinal cellular barrier, allowing harmful *bacterial endotoxins* such as *lipopolysaccharides* (*LPS*) to enter the bloodstream—a process known as *metabolic endotoxemia*. This breach, called *hyperpermeability*, or *leaky gut*, triggers widespread inflammation, affecting everything from cognitive function to cardiovascular health. Time and again, I've seen how restoring gut health can profoundly slow the aging process and promote overall vitality.

Another contributor to inflammation is *metabolic dysfunction*, a condition that becomes increasingly common with advancing age and is discussed in more detail in the next section. Here excess abdominal fat produces those cytokines I just told you about, setting the stage for a vicious cycle of inflammation, metabolic disruption, and tissue damage. This explains why conditions such as insulin resistance (resistance of cells to the effects of insulin) and obesity are tied so closely to chronic diseases and accelerated aging.

The bottom line is this: *inflammation is at the core of aging and age-related diseases*, but it's also a modifiable factor. By addressing its root causes—through targeted lifestyle changes, gut health optimization, and metabolic support—we can break the cycle of inflammaging and reclaim vitality at any age. As we will discuss in chapter 13 on strategies to fight chronic inflammation and gut dysbiosis, in VitalLife I'm implementing latest anti-inflammatory therapies while also drawing from ancient knowledge to manage this menacing inflammation.

The Metabolic Insulin Resistance Theory of Aging

Metabolic dysfunction occurs when the body's systems for managing energy and nutrients break down. If not acted upon, it can progress to *metabolic syndrome*: a cluster of conditions that include high blood sugar, elevated blood pressure, an abnormal cholesterol profile, and excess visceral fat, all of which heighten the risk of diabetes, heart disease, and stroke.

The metabolic insulin resistance theory of aging suggests that as we age, cells become less responsive to insulin, a hormone critical for regulating blood sugar. When insulin can no longer guide glucose effectively into cells, the pancreas compensates by producing more insulin, which eventually exacerbates systemic dysfunction. This reduced sensitivity to insulin disrupts metabolism, accelerates aging, and contributes to diseases. So at its core, poor metabolic health stems from insulin resistance. Estimates suggest that over 90% of Americans are affected by this condition, which can trigger weight gain, elevated blood sugar levels, and a range of serious cardiovascular diseases—including high blood pressure, heart attacks, strokes, and blockages in the arteries of the neck, abdomen, and legs.

Although not always the case, the leading cause of metabolic insulin resistance is *mitochondrial dysfunction*. It entails damage to the tiny powerhouses known as mitochondrial cells that regulate sugar influx—initiating a cycle of reduced cellular energy and declining metabolic dysfunction. We will talk about this further in the following section.

Low-grade inflammation further disrupts metabolism, triggered by refined sugars, processed foods, environmental toxins, and gut dysbiosis. A compromised gut microbiome allows inflammatory endotoxins to circulate, amplifying insulin resistance and metabolic decline. This inflammatory burden creates a *self-reinforcing cycle*: Insulin resistance fuels inflammation, which worsens metabolic dysfunction, hastening aging and age-related conditions. Visceral fat, particularly around the abdomen, stirs up additional trouble by releasing harmful cytokines and cellular factors that damage cells and increase inflammation.

Hormonal imbalances and muscle loss with age also factor into insulin resistance. Declines in growth hormone and testosterone impair glucose management, driving further metabolic decline. Yet there is hope. Integrated clinical approaches we will explore in chapter 12 offer powerful tools to combat insulin resistance and restore metabolic health, providing a path toward healthy aging.

Mitochondrial Energy Theory of Aging

Since my days in medical school, I've been fascinated by the mitochondria, often called the "powerhouses" of cells, the bean-shaped organelles responsible for producing energy in every cell of our body. Mitochondria, with their own DNA, are deeply entwined with the process of aging. They generate *adenosine triphosphate (ATP)*, the energy currency of the cell, through a chemical reaction known as *oxidative phosphorylation*. However, this process also produces harmful byproducts known as *reactive oxygen species* (*ROS*), which can damage cellular components if not neutralized.

Over time, the cumulative exposure to the unstable ROS molecules brings about mutations in the mitochondria's unique DNA (abbreviated mtDNA) and structural damage to the mitochondria themselves. Unlike the nuclear DNA found in a cell's nucleus, mtDNA lacks robust protective proteins called histones and has limited repair mechanisms, making it particularly susceptible to oxidative stress. This damage impairs the mitochondria's ability to produce energy efficiently, leading to a state of dysfunction that accelerates aging.

As discussed above, mitochondrial dysfunction also lies at the heart of insulin resistance. When mitochondria are damaged, receptors on the cell surface refuse to allow blood glucose into the cells despite the presence of high levels of insulin, leaving excessive levels of sugar in the bloodstream. This is the essence of metabolic insulin resistance, a condition that serves as the gateway to a cascade of complications. It's important to clarify here that the cause of insulin resistance is *NOT* refined sugar consumption itself; it stems from mitochondrial damage caused by environmental toxins and a poor diet, particularly one high in fried foods, unhealthy fats, processed products, and excessive calorie intake. Certainly refined sugar can worsen the symptoms of insulin resistance, *but elevated blood sugar is a symptom, not the root cause of insulin resistance.*

> Mitochondrial damage from environmental toxins and an unhealthy diet, particularly one high in fried foods, unhealthy fats, processed products, and excessive calorie intake, is the root cause of insulin resistance and diabetes. High blood sugar is a symptom of a deeper issue.

Mitochondrial dysfunction intricately intertwines with other aging mechanisms, such as inflammation and senescent cells. Deteriorating mitochondria produce more reactive oxygen species, triggering a vicious cycle of cellular damage to proteins, lipids, and DNA. This oxidative stress fuels chronic inflammation, a hidden driver of many age-related diseases. Compounded by inflammation, this leads to complications such as obesity, diabetes, heart disease, and stroke—where high blood sugar is merely a symptom of a deeper, underlying issue.

Gut dysbiosis also plays a critical role in mitochondrial function, which I often address in my clinical practice. Imbalances in gut microbiota disrupt the delicate communication between gut bacteria and mitochondria, increasing ROS production, impairing energy generation, and altering cellular signaling.

Mitochondrial dysfunction also interferes with *apoptosis*—the essential process of removing damaged cells. This allows senescent cells to accumulate in tissues, fueling aging and disease. This dysfunction can manifest in many diseases such as the neurodegenerative disorders Alzheimer's and Parkinson's, where significant mitochondrial damage is evident in affected brain regions, underscoring their central role in disease progression. In cardiovascular diseases, mitochondrial dysfunction in heart cells reduces energy production, contributing to heart failure. In type 2 diabetes, impaired mitochondria in muscle and liver cells decrease insulin sensitivity and glucose uptake. Even sarcopenia, the age-related loss of muscle mass, stems from mitochondrial inefficiency.

To me, this highlights a profound truth: *mitochondria are far more than energy factories*—they are the cornerstone of cellular health, and their decline sets the stage for nearly every hallmark of aging.

Because mitochondria play such a pivotal role, I've made their preservation and restoration a key focus in VitalLife. Strength training, caloric restriction, and emerging therapies such as mitochondrial-targeted treatments and antioxidants are among the approaches I've seen make a real difference in patients' health. As we will discuss in chapter 12, these strategies provide hope for protecting mitochondrial function, potentially slowing the aging process and improving healthspan.

Epigenetics: How Lifestyle and Environment Shape Aging

Genetic and environmental factors also weave their influence into the tapestry of aging. Our genes, the authors of our genetic code, set the foundation for our longevity. However, environmental factors can influence the trajectory of our aging journey. Understanding these factors provides us with the knowledge to sway this dance in our favor, promoting a healthier, longer life.

I know most of us think of our genetic makeup as a fixed blueprint for how we age, but epigenetics tells a different story. While your DNA remains the same throughout your life, how your genes are *expressed*—in other words, how they really function— can change. The word *epigenetics* refers to the molecular switches that turn genes on or off, influenced by factors such as diet, emotional stress, lifestyle, and environmental toxins such as pesticides, chemicals, and pollutants. These switches don't change the genetic code itself, but they do alter how your cells read that code, affecting everything from your metabolism, to how efficiently your cells repair themselves. *Epigenetic modifications*—the subtle adjustments to our genetic expression—influence which genes are turned on or off, thereby dictating the process of aging.

These epigenetic changes accumulate over time. This contributes to everything from wrinkles and loss of muscle tone to more serious age-related diseases like cancer, cardiovascular disease, and cognitive decline.

> Our genetic code is not set in stone; we can influence it by choices we make every day regarding our lifestyle, diet, and personalized health strategies. So we do have the power to change how we age—or don't age.

While we can't rewrite our genetic code, we know how informed choices can significantly influence genetic expression and, consequently, our aging trajectory. It is exciting to see how this understanding transforms patients' perspectives—*from feeling genetically predetermined to becoming active participants in their longevity journey.*

Now that we've explored the biological foundations of aging, it's time to put all this science together. In the next chapter, I describe what I believe is a paradigm shift in conventional thinking of aging and how this new perspective replaces outdated ones, thus allowing for a better understanding of disease formation and progression, and the development of innovative treatment programs such as VitalLife.

CHAPTER 6

A Disease Called Aging

Doctors are men who prescribe medicines of which they know little, to cure diseases of which they know less, for human beings of whom they know nothing.
—*Voltaire, French writer and philosopher (1694–1778)*

Do not go where the path may lead, go instead where there is no path and leave a trail.
—*Ralph Waldo Emerson, American writer (1803–1882)*

Steve, fifty-six years old, is a successful chiropractic physician with multiple offices and more than fifty employees, including several chiropractors, physical therapists, and physician assistants. A few years back, he was diagnosed with high blood pressure (hypertension), mild obesity, diabetes, high cholesterol, and erectile dysfunction. Despite regular appointments with his primary care physician and various specialists every two or three months, and despite following all of his doctors' advice, he continued to have difficulty managing his medical conditions.

He was repeatedly told by his heart, diabetes, kidney, and eye specialists that, despite their best treatments and interventions, they could not cure any of his diseases. The most they could do was slow their progression and delay complications such as heart attack, stroke, kidney failure, and eye damage (retinopathy), which would ultimately lead to premature death.

Steve felt utterly powerless and crushed by dejection, trapped in a despair so overwhelming that hope and a way forward seemed completely out of reach.

> He was told repeatedly by his specialists that they cannot cure any of his diseases. The best they can do is delay the eventual complications including heart attack, retinopathy, kidney failure, and premature death.

No one ever told him that all of his medical issues shared a common origin. It is called *atherosclerosis*, the formation of fatty plaques in the arteries that carry oxygen-laden blood cells throughout the body. *Beginning as early as our teenage years*, the buildup of deposits on the vessels' inner lining gradually narrows the pathway through which blood accesses all organs. If an artery becomes completely obstructed, the blood-starved tissue may sustain damage or even die.

We will discuss more about this condition later in this chapter; as we'll see, atherosclerosis is very common, *affecting about half of Americans over the age of forty-five*, but most people are unaware of it and few specialists discuss this with their patients because they specialize in the diseases of their organ system only. The sooner we tackle atherosclerosis, the sooner we can change the course of all those common diseases and we might even help cure them. When we understand atherosclerosis as the root cause of so many common diseases as we age, we can unlock the secret to unclogging these arteries and get real treatment.

By addressing his atherosclerosis with a personalized VitalLife program, Steve started to lose weight and gain more control over his blood pressure, blood sugar, and cholesterol levels. He also saw improvement in his energy levels and strength, as well as in his biomarkers. Soon his cholesterol levels were within normal range without any medicines. He was also able to reduce the dosages of the diabetes and blood pressure medications that he had been taking prior to seeing me.

The Aging Triad and Cellular Feedback Loop

Now let's delve into what my experience over these decades has taught me about the key cellular processes of why we really age and what causes the diseases of aging. I believe that aging does not stem from one single, solitary cause. While we often segment different processes, organs, and systems to study them in isolation, the body operates as a single *whole*. What's more, these processes amplify one another in the *cellular feedback loop*. It's a mesmerizing, complex interplay of several processes that you read about in the previous chapter. Each process affects the others, fueling a downward spiral that accelerates aging, disease, and an overall decline in health.

I've been particularly captivated by the interplay of metabolic insulin resistance, chronic inflammation, and mitochondrial dysfunction, or what I've come to call the *Aging Triad*. Although they are three distinct cellular processes, these partners in crime conspire to form a sophisticated network, compounding their harmful effects on your health. I've explained how inflammatory cascades can trigger insulin resistance while simultaneously compromising mitochondrial function, triggering a self-perpetuating cycle of cellular aging.

What excites me most is knowing that these mechanisms are not simply time-driven deteriorations—they are dynamic systems that we can influence and, in some cases, even reverse.

> **The VitalLife Aging Triad**
> It consists of three key cellular processes—mitochondrial dysfunction, metabolic insulin resistance, and systemic chronic low-grade inflammation—that interact closely with one another in a cellular feedback loop and are instrumental in causing aging and diseases of aging.

I believe, and science is pointing more and more in this direction, that while other cellular processes contributing to aging are important, the most significant factor in aging and chronic diseases is *chronic inflammation*. Also, an improving picture of how inflammation modulates metabolism provides us with a new perspective for using anti-inflammatory strategies to correct the metabolic consequences. In 1876 an esteemed German physician named Wilhelm Ebstein concluded that sodium salicylate, a chemical compound similar to aspirin, could make the symptoms of diabetes mellitus totally disappear. More than a hundred years ago, high doses of salicylates were shown to lower glucose levels in diabetic patients. Furthermore high-dose salicylates appear to improve cardiometabolic risk factors in healthy individuals and in type 2 diabetes patients. Also, high-dose aspirin, colchicine (a gout inflammation medicine), and a low dose of an opiate antagonist called naltrexone help to decrease atherosclerosis blockages. Scientists have shown that infliximab, a monoclonal antibody medication used to treat certain inflammatory and autoimmune diseases, was able to reduce inflammation in atherosclerosis by blocking the pro-inflammatory cytokine known as tumor necrosis factor-alpha (TNF-α).

Impairment of mitochondrial function is another piece of this puzzle of aging. It is caused by environmental toxins, unhealthy fats, refined sugars, and an excessive workload on these cellular powerhouses from simply eating too many calories in our Western diet. When mitochondria are damaged, this also leads to insulin resistance, a condition that serves as the gateway to a cascade of complications. Mitochondrial dysfunction also interweaves with other aging mechanisms, such as chronic inflammation, senescence cells, and epigenetics.

As we discussed in detail in the previous chapter, systemic chronic inflammation fuels this metabolic and mitochondrial dysfunction further, producing a vicious cycle. Insulin resistance doesn't just bring about elevated blood sugar—it is the precursor to a host of life-threatening conditions, including obesity, type 2 diabetes, heart disease, atherosclerosis, and stroke. And yet the primary culprit here isn't sugar itself; it's the mitochondria being overwhelmed by toxins, unhealthy fats, and an excessive workload. High blood sugar is merely a symptom of this deeper, systemic issue.

I've often questioned why so many physicians worldwide are laser-focused solely on controlling blood sugar levels with insulin and anti-diabetes medications, while neglecting to treat the root cause of insulin resistance. Yes, lowering blood sugar may slow the progression of complications—slightly—but it's like bailing water from a sinking boat without fixing the leak.

> Chronic diseases such as diabetes, heart disease, and stroke are *diseases of choice*—entirely **PREVENTABLE** and **REVERSIBLE** with the proper lifestyle changes and health strategies.

Sadly, I've seen too many patients with diabetes diligently follow their physicians' advice to the letter, only to endure perpetual devastating complications: kidney failure, nerve damage, heart attack, stroke, and eventually premature death. Through VitalLife, my mission is to shift the focus away from merely chasing blood sugar numbers and toward addressing the true root causes of insulin resistance.

The VitalLife Model of Aging

So, how does the aging process really start? Whether it is aging or any of the related chronic diseases, I have put together a comprehensive scientific model that I call the VitalLife Model of Aging.

Aging begins with the interplay of epigenetics and environmental factors (processed food, fried food, unhealthy fats, excessive caloric intake, smoking, alcohol, toxins, allergens, emotional stress, and chemicals). This is the ideal place to start and make a real impact on health—prevention at all costs. When not addressed—sadly, that is true for most of us—this leads to the Aging Triad of systemic chronic inflammation, mitochondrial dysfunction, and metabolic insulin resistance.

These three processes then amplify one another and cause cell dysfunction, senescent cells, sarcopenia, and atherosclerosis in the entire body, which leads to a disease process of aging. High blood sugar, high cholesterol, high blood pressure, and diseases such as heart attack, stroke, diabetes, retinopathy, kidney failure, Alzheimer's, and arthritis *are only aftereffects of the aging process. The root cause of disease and aging is this Aging Triad.* That's why addressing the underlying factors of the Aging Triad becomes crucial for restoring health, curing disease, and slowing the pace of aging.

> **Aging starts with the interplay of epigenetics and environmental factors:**
> processed food, fried food, unhealthy fats, excessive caloric intake, smoking, alcohol, toxins, allergens, stress, chemicals. Our priority must be to end America's epidemic of chronic illnesses by emphasizing healthy food and the elimination of environmental toxins.

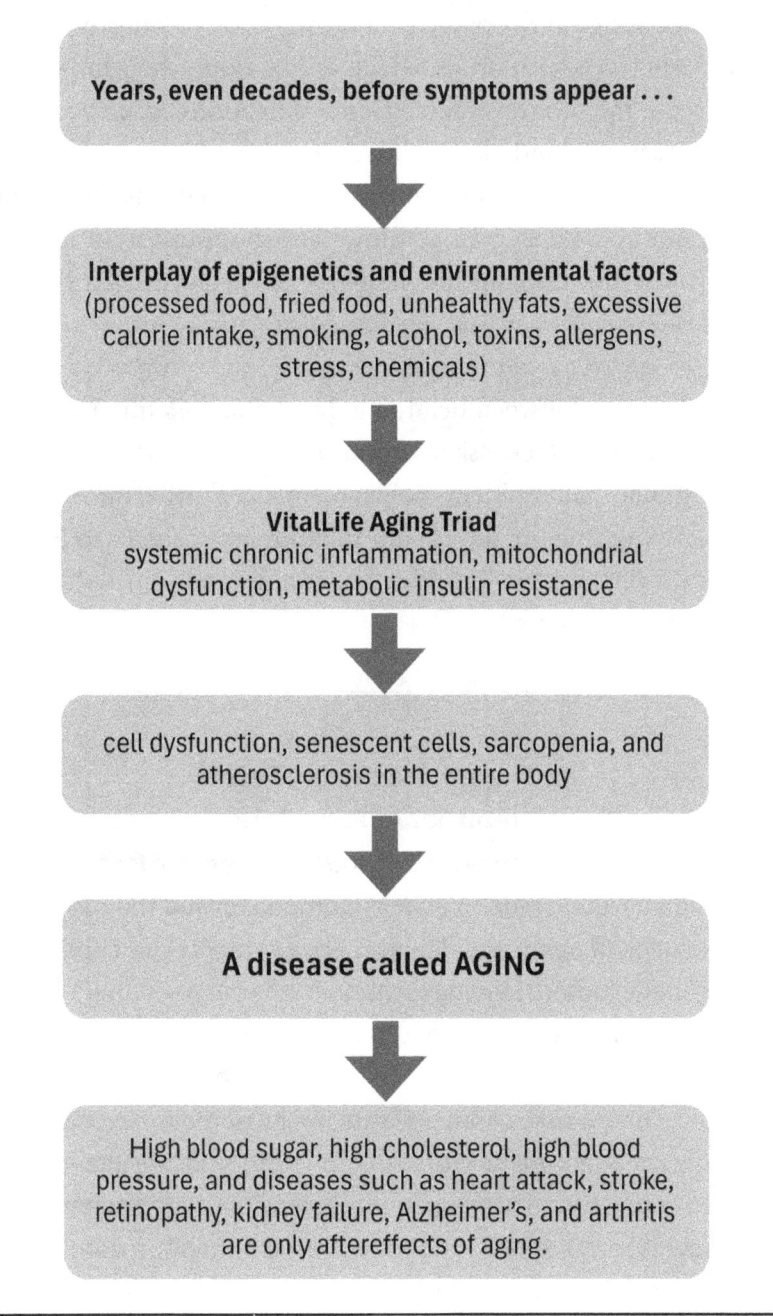

As you can see, the Aging Triad is the most important issue regarding aging as well as most of the common diseases. Instead of physicians focusing on decreasing blood sugar or blood pressure or cholesterol levels with drugs, which are no doubt very important to decrease the progression of the complications, *we all must focus on the root cause* behind all the suffering.

While reducing high blood sugar with pills or insulin in diabetic patients and decreasing low-density lipoprotein cholesterol with statins remains the mainstay of cardiovascular disease treatment, the *attenuation of systemic inflammation is now emerging as a target of interest, especially in patients with recurrent heart attack events.* The association between heightened systemic inflammation and increased heart attack risk is supported by several large clinical, observational, and epidemiological studies. Furthermore, clinical trials exploring the use of anti-inflammatory agents to inhibit systemic inflammation have demonstrated significant reductions in heart attack events.

An Urgent Plea to My Fellow Healthcare Providers

Now that the science is clear, the time has come for physicians worldwide to shift their focus toward the root causes of aging and disease. Environmental and epigenetic factors leading to chronic inflammation, mitochondrial dysfunction, and metabolic insulin resistance are at the heart of aging and chronic diseases.

For the sake of our patients, we must move beyond the knee-jerk reaction of merely trying to fix lab results—lowering blood pressure, cholesterol, or blood sugar levels in isolation. Instead, we need to adopt a comprehensive, root-cause approach that truly restores healing, cures disease, and extends both healthspan and lifespan.

Biological Aging Is a Treatable Disease

What was once seen as an inevitable decline can now be understood as a modifiable biological process. Just like diabetes or heart disease, aging has identifiable causes—and, remarkably, potential treatments. As we've explored, aging is driven by precise molecular and cellular processes that can be measured, monitored, and even modified. Mechanisms such as chronic inflammation, insulin resistance, cellular senescence, and mitochondrial dysfunction, long thought to be unavoidable, are now actionable targets for intervention.

While the science behind these processes is complex, the message is simple and empowering: aging isn't merely the passage of time; rather it is shaped by our biology and the choices we make. The best part? With targeted interventions, many of these processes can not only be slowed but also, in some cases, reversed, offering new hope for a healthier, more vibrant future.

> According to the VitalLife model, aging is nothing but a biological process caused by modifiable external factors, rather than an immutable program written in stone by nature. Aging, therefore, is a disease of choice, one that can be prevented and reversed.

This shift in understanding aging as a biological process rather than an immutable program is groundbreaking. With diagnostic criteria, measurable biomarkers, and targeted therapies, we can tackle aging like any other medical condition. Instead of merely managing diseases such as Alzheimer's, arthritis, and cardiovascular conditions, we can address their root cause: *aging itself.*

Atherosclerosis: The Silent Driver of Aging and Disease

Now that we've discussed the primary reasons behind aging and chronic diseases, let's turn our attention to the atherosclerosis affecting millions of Americans, including Steve, the patient you met at the beginning of this chapter. People are often diagnosed with various conditions affecting specific organs—such as heart attacks, strokes, eye damage, or kidney failure—and these are treated as separate diseases by specialists. *Yet all of these issues stem from this single underlying condition that simply manifests in one organ first.*

Wouldn't it make more sense to treat this systemic condition with a whole-body approach, rather than focusing solely on one organ—such as performing coronary balloon angioplasties (a procedure to widen blocked or narrowed arteries) for the heart while neglecting the health of other organs? This fragmented approach does great disservice to our patients, undermining the whole-person care they deserve.

Atherosclerosis, often referred to as *vascular aging*, is the common culprit. In this condition, your arteries—the body's vital transportation system—*become narrowed and hardened* due to plaque buildup. This lack of blood flow impairs cellular function and accelerates the aging processes across tissues and organs leading to chest pain, heart attacks, blindness, strokes, or kidney damage, depending on where the problem occurs.

Here's something crucial I've observed in my practice: aging is about what's silently happening in your blood vessels throughout your body, in every organ. This vascular aging may be the major driver—*or even the final step*—that leads to aging and the diseases associated with it. To truly understand the aging process, we must grasp the cellular and functional changes occurring in the vasculature over time.

Imagine your arteries as tunnels. With age, the opening, or *lumen*, can narrow due to the accumulation of plaques on the inner walls. The vessels also lose some of their elasticity. When this happens, it's as if your blood gets marooned in traffic jams throughout your body. Organs and tissues are starved of the oxygen and nutrients they need, especially during high-demand periods such as exercise or stress.

As we have discussed, what's especially alarming is that atherosclerosis doesn't wait until old age to present. The process *starts as early as the teenage years*, highlighting just how early vascular dysfunction can begin to take root. Recognizing this early onset underscores the importance of taking proactive measures to prevent and address this systemic condition.

While atherosclerosis begins silently as early as adolescence, it is deeply consequential. Fatty streaks, then plaques—a mix of cholesterol, fatty substances, cellular waste, the mineral *calcium*, and *fibrin*, a fibrous substance essential for stopping bleeding from an injury—embed themselves in the artery walls. This buildup, triggered by damage to the *endothelium* (the delicate inner lining), reduces blood flow and sets the stage for some of the most serious health problems, including heart attack, stroke, and peripheral artery disease.

So, why does this damage occur? A multitude of factors such as genetics, environmental factors, and your lifestyle, including consumption of ultra-processed foods and fried foods, smoking, drinking alcohol, stress, and gut dysbiosis all lead to systemic chronic inflammation. Inflammation in the endothelium, the inner lining of the blood vessels, causes it to break down. And now research is showing that the major regulator in diet is oxidized "bad oil" LDL (*oxLDL*), which is ruthlessly inflammatory in nature. The special immune cells called macrophages engulf this oxLDL in an effort to remove it and become special "foam cells" that trigger multiple pathways that lead to endothelium damage. Once damaged, the endothelium becomes a magnet for cholesterol and other substances in the blood, forming sticky plaques that grow and harden over time. These plaques not only narrow the arteries but also destabilize, potentially rupturing and triggering blood clots that can completely block blood flow, causing serious conditions such as stroke and heart attack.

All scientists and clinicians stand on the shoulders of great men who came before us. A little historical perspective will be helpful here. Egyptian papyri from almost five thousand years ago refer to heat and redness as concomitants of disease. In the first century AD, the Roman physician and encyclopedist Aulus Cornelius Celsus astutely defined the cardinal signs of inflammation: redness, swelling, heat, and pain. In fact, in 1856 a German pathologist named Rudolf Virchow was the first proponent of the hypothesis that "Atherosclerosis is an inflammatory disease" (*endarteritis chronica deformans*, meaning "chronic inflammation of internal arteries leading to deformation"). In 1999 another pathologist, American Russell Ross, published a landmark paper in the *New England Journal of Medicine* in which he proposed for the first time that atherosclerosis was definitively an inflammatory disease. Furthermore, it did not result simply from lipid accumulation, as had been thought previously.

Atherosclerosis Is a Systemic Condition That Impacts the Entire Body

Although its symptoms may first appear in one area, such as a heart attack or stroke, atherosclerosis is much more than just a localized condition. It is a systemic process that silently *impacts arteries throughout the entire body*, becoming a driving force behind both aging and the diseases associated with it. Often called a "silent killer," it progresses quietly until significant symptoms or complications arise.

However, there is good news: *Atherosclerosis is both preventable and manageable.* Addressing root causes—by overhauling diet, reducing inflammation, addressing mitochondrial dysfunction, removing toxins, and improving the gut microbiome—can slow or even reverse its progression. Multiple studies, especially those from the Cleveland Clinic, one of the top academic medical centers in the country, have shown that adopting healthy habits can yield significant improvements in blockages in the heart arteries, weight management, blood pressure, and levels of cholesterol and sugar. What's more, even patients with severe coronary artery blockages can see improved blood flow, possibly eliminating the need for invasive surgery.

> Treating the root causes of atherosclerosis—by improving diet, reducing inflammation, addressing mitochondrial dysfunction, removing toxins, and improving the gut microbiome—can slow or even reverse its progression.

In short, atherosclerosis is far more than just "clogged arteries." It is a progressive disease of the entire vascular system. Understanding that it is rooted in the interplay of lifestyle, environment, and biology—and acting early—are crucial to preventing its devastating effects and preserving your long-term health.

The takeaway is simple: if you provide your body with the right conditions, it has an incredible ability to heal itself. In that sense, diabetes, heart disease, stroke, and even biological aging are diseases of choice—entirely preventable and reversible with the proper lifestyle changes and health strategies.

A Special Note About Heart Disease

Now, let's talk about the most common medical condition affecting Americans and the leading cause of death in the United States: heart disease. This topic is personal to me because I've seen too many lives cut short by *this disease that is both preventable and reversible*. When I think about the staggering number of people affected each year and the immense resources spent on this disease, I feel frustrated because *it is not something we have to accept as inevitable.*

And, ominously, since 2019, heart disease has been fast becoming more common in the younger population, due to Millennials' and Gen Zers' penchant for indulging in processed and ultra-processed foods, unhealthy fats, low-fiber foods, vaping, and alcohol and drug use, as well as their sedentary lifestyle compounded by an increased incidence of obesity, high blood pressure, stress, loneliness, and diabetes.

According to the US Centers for Disease Control and Prevention (CDC), one in two men and one in three women in the United States will develop heart disease during their lifetime. Let that sink in for a moment. And, each year, over 700,000 people in United States lose their lives to heart disease in U.S., according to the CDC. The cost of managing this disease exceeds $300 billion annually.

Coronary heart disease (CHD) is the most common type of heart disease. It is primarily caused by blockages in the arteries, a condition we discussed earlier known as atherosclerosis. Every year, more than 800,000 Americans suffer a heart attack—one every 40 seconds—resulting in approximately 375,000 deaths. To put this into perspective, it's the equivalent of two 747 jumbo jets, each carrying 500 passengers, crashing every single day in the United States. Imagine the outrage and urgency such a daily tragedy would spark—yet we quietly endure this type of loss from CHD. It's heartbreaking to realize that with the right knowledge and action, countless lives could be saved. This preventable suffering serves as a powerful, urgent call to act and change the course for millions.

A famous 1998 study known as the China Study, conducted by Cornell University and Oxford University in partnership with the Chinese government, surveyed a population of about a half million people in China's rural Guizhou Province in the 1980s. Their diets (*low in fat and high in dietary fiber and plant foods*) were in sharp contrast to the calorie-rich animal-based diets of Western countries. The results, published in 2004 by nutritional biochemist T. Colin Campbell, PhD, were striking: over a three-year period, not one death from coronary artery disease was reported in men over age sixty-five. *That's correct: NONE.*

Similarly, research from the 1950s in Japan found heart disease to be incredibly rare. But here's the catch: when people from countries such as China, Japan, and India *immigrated to the United States and adopted the typical American diet and lifestyle*, their rates of heart disease and stroke quickly matched—and sometimes exceeded—those of native-born Americans. I've seen this firsthand with patients and my family members, and it's a sobering reminder of how powerful our lifestyle choices can be.

As I said earlier, here's something that is significant but most people don't know: *atherosclerosis begins in childhood*. I find that fact deeply motivating to share with others, especially for the welfare of our children. One study from 1953, published in the *Journal of the American Medical Association* (*JAMA*), changed everything we thought we knew about heart disease. It analyzed three hundred autopsies of Americans who had died in the Korean War, with an average age of just twenty-two. A shocking 77 percent already exhibited signs of atherosclerosis in their arteries, with some of the blockages exceeding 90 percent. Can you imagine? In people barely out of their teens? That hit me hard the first time I read it.

It gets worse. In the 1980s, researchers studied young accident victims aged three to twenty-six. By the age of *ten*, many already had fatty streaks—the earliest stage of atherosclerosis—in their arteries. By the time they were in their twenties, these streaks had progressed to full-blown plaques, as seen in the *JAMA* study. When I talk to my patients, I often tell them, "Heart disease isn't just a disease of old age. It's a disease of childhood showing up in the adult years."

> Heart disease is *not* a disease of old age. It is a disease of childhood showing up in the adult years. Science is clear: it is a disease of choice and is completely preventable and even reversible.

Here's the real tragedy: *people are almost always diagnosed too late.* By the time symptoms appear, such as chest pain or shortness of breath, the damage has already been building up for decades. The typical treatments include medications, angioplasty, or coronary artery bypass surgery. These interventions can only provide relief to symptoms. *But they do nothing to cure the disease. And, sadly, any relief in symptoms fades with time,* so patients end up undergoing repeated angioplasties and bypass surgeries. I've seen this over and over with so many people in my forty years as physician, and it's one of the reasons I'm so passionate about educating people about this entirely PREVENTABLE and REVERSIBLE disease.

And let's be honest: the financial incentives in our healthcare system don't help. Cardiologists, hospitals, and healthcare companies profit immensely from these expensive procedures. Did you know that the United States, despite having just 5 percent of the world's population, performs more than half of the globe's heart surgeries and procedures? We spend more than $300 billion annually treating symptoms—but comparatively little educating the public on how to eradicate heart disease altogether.

This is so significant that I feel compelled to reiterate here: there's hope because heart disease doesn't have to be a death sentence. It doesn't even have to happen in the first place. Atherosclerosis and heart disease are not only *preventable*—they're *reversible*. Heart disease has a cause. It doesn't just appear out of nowhere. And if it has a cause, it has a solution. Here's the bottom line: *heart disease is a disease of choice*—its primary driver being our diet and lifestyle. By adopting specific dietary changes, making lifestyle modifications, and following a few simple strategies—which we'll discuss in the pages ahead—you can take control of your health and even reverse this disease. I've seen it happen and I'm here to show you how.

Sarcopenia: A Common Condition You've Probably Never Heard of

Sarcopenia (from the Greek: *sarx* for flesh, *penia* for loss) might be one of the most dangerous and common conditions related to aging and age-related diseases that you've probably never heard of. It refers to the *gradual loss of muscle mass, strength, and function—a hallmark of aging that can begin as early as your forties* and accelerates with time. In my clinical experience, I've seen how sarcopenia profoundly impacts people's lives, particularly folks in their sixties and beyond, leaving them frail, less mobile, and more vulnerable to falls and fractures.

But *sarcopenia doesn't just shrink muscle size, it also undermines muscle quality* by weakening the muscle fibers, rendering muscle contractions less efficient and compromising the muscle's self-repair mechanism, increasing the time it takes to recover from even minor injuries.

Sarcopenia is a complex, multifaceted process caused by interconnected biological and lifestyle factors. Addressing and understanding these root causes is crucial for preventing and managing the condition effectively.

A key factor in sarcopenia's development is *anabolic resistance*, where the body's ability to build and repair muscle in response to protein intake and exercise diminishes. It is often seen as early as in your forties. Here muscle cells become less responsive to the signals from anabolic hormones such as testosterone, even in females, leaving muscles unable to synthesize protein as efficiently as they once did.

Understanding and addressing anabolic resistance is critical because it impairs muscle maintenance and regeneration, accelerating muscle loss and increasing the risk of frailty and reduced mobility, and worsening chronic diseases such as cardiovascular diseases, diabetes, and kidney disease.

At the cellular level, sarcopenia is closely linked to *mitochondrial dysfunction*. With decreasing efficiency as we age, mitochondrial energy production declines, making it harder for muscle cells to perform and regenerate. Additionally, increased oxidative stress brings out more of those pesky reactive oxygen species, which damage cellular proteins and DNA, further impairing muscle function.

Hormonal changes, too, play a critical role. With age, levels of anabolic (protein building) hormones such as testosterone, growth hormone (GH), and *insulin-like growth factor-1 (IGF-1)* decline. These hormones are essential for muscle protein synthesis and repair. Simultaneously, there is an increase in *catabolic* (protein breakdown) hormones like *cortisol*—the stress hormone—which can accelerate muscle breakdown.

Chronic inflammation contributes significantly to sarcopenia. Elevated levels of pro-inflammatory cytokines such as *interleukin-6 (IL-6)* and TNF-α interfere with muscle protein synthesis, reduce satellite cell activity (a key to muscle repair), and promote muscle protein degradation. This low-grade systemic inflammation is exacerbated by conditions such as insulin resistance and obesity, and a sedentary lifestyle.

Another critical factor is the *decline in neuromuscular function*. With advancing years, we incur a loss of *motor neurons*, the nerve supplying the muscles. This results in fewer and less effective signals to muscles, contributing to muscle weakness and atrophy. *Diet and lifestyle* also play significant roles in causing sarcopenia. Inadequate protein intake, essential for muscle maintenance, is a common issue among older adults. *Combined with physical inactivity*, which accelerates muscle loss, these factors create a feedback loop of declining muscle function and increased frailty. Finally, sarcopenia is also compounded by *medical conditions* such as diabetes, cardiovascular disease, and other chronic illnesses, all of which impair the body's ability to maintain muscle mass and strength.

As you can see, this dangerous sarcopenia is driven by a combination of multiple factors and accelerates the process of aging. Addressing these underlying causes through targeted interventions can prevent or even reverse muscle loss, making it a key focus of the VitalLife program for healthy aging and longevity. I will discuss the treatment strategies to combat this in chapter 12.

The Time to Act Is Now

Now that we've explored the biological foundations of aging and its associated chronic diseases, it is time to act. Whether you're looking to undo the effects of aging, reverse diseases, optimize your health, or simply feel more alive, I'll guide you through everything you need to know to unlock your own full potential. You are now ready to take the first steps toward a healthier, stronger, and more vibrant future.

I must emphasize an important clinical point: many of these advanced regenerative therapies discussed in the following chapters require careful patient selection and precise administration. Some treatments discussed in subsequent sections have specific safety considerations; limited availability in certain regions, forcing patients to travel to outside the United States; significant financial considerations; and require administration by physicians with extensive experience in regenerative protocols. The complexity of these interventions demands careful customization based on individual health parameters and therapeutic goals.

In the next chapter, we will talk about the first step in your journey toward a healthier, more vibrant, longer life: to assess your current state of health. By testing key biomarkers and analyzing your genetics, we can uncover the unique factors affecting your own health and aging process. This provides a clear road map for how to tailor the VitalLife program to your individual needs, optimizing your energy, performance, and longevity.

PART 3

THE VITALLIFE PROGRAM FOR A YOUNGER AND VIBRANT YOU

CHAPTER 7

A Personalized Assessment: Biomarkers and DNA Tests

What gets measured gets managed.
—Peter Drucker, Austrian American economist (1909–2005)

Without data, you're just another
person with an opinion.
—W. Edwards Deming, American expert in business
management (1900–1993)

In the quest to optimize your health and extend your vitality, the first step is understanding where you stand today. No two people age the same way, and that's why personalized testing is at the core of this program. Gone are the days of one-size-fits-all approaches to health.

Biomarkers are biological indicators that indicate the state of your cells, organs, and body. These can be measured and used to diagnose and monitor health, disease, and aging. By leveraging advanced testing methods—such as biomarkers, DNA biological age assessments, and cancer screenings—we can gain a clear, individualized picture of your current health status.

Think of biomarkers as your body's way of telling its unique story: they're the vital signs of your aging journey that we carefully listen to together. I've come to appreciate that these sophisticated measurements are like a map, showing us exactly where your body is on its path to optimal health and longevity, and enabling us to craft a plan that is uniquely yours, combining cutting-edge regenerative medicine with time-tested healing wisdom.

> **VitalLife Biomarker Blueprint**
> It is a unique aging signature of your cell function, created by measuring key personalized biomarkers and your DNA biological age.

In my practice, I've developed a detailed VitalLife Biomarker Blueprint. It includes an extensive battery of biomarkers and genetic factors that can be personalized to identify each person's unique aging signature. This comprehensive testing reveals your own specific biological age accelerators. Through years of clinical experience, I've found that understanding these individual patterns is crucial for optimizing healthspan and vitality for each person. I've learned through years of clinical practice that therapeutic success is critically dependent on this precise personalization targeted to a person's unique biology to improve biological age as well as lifespan.

Also, I find it very important is to repeat these tests at regular intervals to minimize any risks of treatments, assess the progress, and modify the personalized program if needed. By systematically tracking these key markers, we're not making educated guesses—we're making informed, science-backed decisions about your health. We can see, with remarkable precision, how each intervention is contributing to your journey toward enhanced vitality and longevity.

Biomarkers and DNA Tests

This section outlines some of the core tests that form the foundation of a personalized anti-aging strategy.

Hormonal and vitamin levels are key indicators of aging. Hormones such as testosterone, estradiol, follicle-stimulating hormone (FSH), luteinizing hormone (LH), thyroid hormones, cortisol, and prolactin tend to decline with advancing years, affecting energy, muscle mass, sleep, and sexual function. Levels of the hormone dehydroepiandrosterone (DHEA), too, drop with age, which is linked to cognitive decline and bone density loss. Monitoring growth hormone and IGF-1 levels is equally important, as lower levels contribute to reducing skin elasticity, muscle mass, strength, and overall vitality. Vitamin levels, particularly D_3, B_{12}, folic acid, and homocysteine also provide insights into metabolic health and nutrient absorption.

Biological age is measured through telomere (protective caps at the ends of chromosomes that are made of DNA and protein) length and DNA methylation patterns. DNA methylation is an epigenetic mark that adds a methyl group to DNA, which can regulate gene expression. This gives us a deeper understanding of how well your body is aging at the cellular level. Shorter telomeres are linked to a higher risk of age-related diseases, while DNA methylation can reveal how old your body truly is in relation to your chronological age. These tests help in tailoring a program to slow down cellular aging and address any areas of concern that may accelerate the aging process.

Oxidative stress tests are vital in assessing the damage caused by free radicals. For example, levels of malondialdehyde (MDA), a byproduct of lipid peroxidation, rise with increased oxidative damage, and 8-hydroxy-2′deoxyguanosine (abbreviated, thankfully, 8-OHdG), an indicator of oxidative DNA damage, is elevated in aging and disease. Monitoring these helps determine the level of oxidative stress and allows interventions to support antioxidant defense systems.

Metabolic and cardiovascular markers provide a window into your metabolic health and cardiovascular risk. Instead of body-mass index (BMI) which assesses your weight relative to height, it is more accurate to check waist-to-height ratio (WtHR), that focuses on the distribution of body fat, specifically abdominal fat, by comparing waist circumference to height. WtHR is now considered a stronger indicator of the risk of developing cardiovascular disease.

Tracking fasting insulin, c-peptide, leptin, and glucose levels, hemoglobin A1c, and insulin sensitivity through tests such as Homeostasis Model Assessment for Insulin Resistance (HOMA-IR) helps us to understand how well your body manages blood sugar and energy. To calculate HOMA-IR at home, you'll need your fasting blood glucose (mg/dL) and fasting insulin levels (mU/L), then use this simple formula: (fasting glucose x fasting insulin) divided by 405. Less than 1 means you are insulin-sensitive, greater than 1.9 indicates early insulin resistance, and greater than 2.9 indicates significant insulin resistance.

For all my patients, even if they are not diagnosed with diabetes, I use continuous glucose monitors (CGMs), which track glucose in real time and offer even deeper insights into metabolic function and insulin resistance.

Additionally, a lipid profile, including total cholesterol, LDL, HDL, triglycerides, and high-sensitivity C-reactive protein (hs-CRP), assesses cardiovascular risk. Advanced blood tests to determine your levels of LDL particle size and pattern, oxidized LDL, lipoprotein (a), apolipoprotein B (ApoB), and apolipoprotein A1 (Apo A-1) provide a more detailed picture of heart health and, I believe, a more accurate assessment of cardiac risks than traditional good- and bad-cholesterol tests.

For all my patients, I target for a total cholesterol level of less than 150 milligrams per deciliter of blood (abbreviated mg/dl) and an LDL (bad cholesterol) level under 70 mg/dl. It is a more aggressive approach than that recommended by the American Heart Association.

Mitochondrial function is another key aspect of aging. As we age, our mitochondria become less efficient and produce less energy. Measuring ATP levels and mitochondrial DNA mutations provides a clear picture of mitochondrial health, helping guide interventions to support cellular energy and vitality.

Hematological (blood) tests and organ-specific tests, such as complete blood counts, electrolyte levels, and tests of liver and kidney function, are also important for overall health.

Cognitive function assessments are vital for understanding brain health. Evaluating memory, attention, and executive functions for planning, organizing, and decision-making skills helps identify any signs of cognitive decline and informs strategies to protect and enhance brain function. These tests are crucial for creating personalized brain health plans for patients who are at risk or who already exhibit cognitive and memory decline, especially in patients with brain injuries, Alzheimer's, and Parkinson's disease.

Genetic cancer screening has advanced significantly with tests such as one called Galleri, which can detect more than fifty types of cancer early. This revolutionary blood test looks for abnormal patterns in DNA that are associated with cancer, allowing for earlier intervention in malignancies that typically go undetected until late stages.

Peak performance tests such as VO2max (maximal oxygen consumption, the highest amount of oxygen a person can utilize during intense exercise), body composition analysis, and isokinetic strength testing provide insights into cardiovascular fitness, muscle mass, and physical power. These assessments are especially useful for athletes but can be beneficial for anyone looking to optimize physical performance as they age.

Grip strength test measures how much force a person can squeeze with their hand. It is a measure of the muscular strength of one's forearm muscles. Research indicates that it can help assess age-related decline, heart health, and athletic performance. It is typically performed using a hand-held dynamometer, but it can also be measured with a weight scale.

Medical Technological devices, or MedTech as they're often called, are useful in monitoring markers and function. The ones I use most often include the Libre3 continuous glucose monitor for insulin resistance, which is helpful even in patients without diabetes, as well as Oura, Apple Watch, EMAY Sleep O2 Pulse Ox (to screen for sleep apnea, even in thin people with few specific symptoms, such as daytime snoozing), KardiaMobile (for *atrial fibrillation*, a condition in which the upper chambers of the heart beat rapidly and out of rhythm, causing symptoms such as palpitations, lightheadedness, shortness of breath, and chest pain), and the Wellue O2 Ring pulse oximeter to calculate the oxygen saturation of a person's arterial blood.

Together these biomarkers and devices offer a comprehensive view of an individual's health and aging process, guiding personalized interventions that are tailored to slow aging and enhance overall vitality and promote healthspan. Regular testing and monitoring help assess progress and refine strategies in anti-aging efforts.

Chronic Inflammation Diagnostic Testing

Chronic inflammation is a key cause of numerous medical concerns, including metabolic dysfunction, cardiovascular disease, autoimmune disorders, and aging-related conditions. Here are some of the specific tests that I rely on for identifying, monitoring, and gaining valuable insights into a patient's underlying inflammation:

- **White Blood Cell (WBC) Count:** A high WBC count can indicate systemic inflammation or infection, reflecting the body's immune response.
- **C3 and C4 Complements:** These proteins are part of the immune system's complement pathway; elevated or decreased levels can signal inflammation or autoimmune activity.
- **High-Sensitivity C-Reactive Protein (hs-CRP):** A sensitive marker for low-grade inflammation, often linked to cardiovascular risk and chronic conditions.
- **Ferritin:** While primarily a measure of iron storage, elevated ferritin levels can indicate inflammation or oxidative stress.
- **Fibrinogen:** A blood-clotting factor that increases during inflammation and is associated with higher risks of cardiovascular disease and stroke.
- **Lipoprotein-Associated Phospholipase A2 (Lp-PLA2):** A marker of blood vessel inflammation, useful in assessing cardiovascular disease risk.
- **Tumor Necrosis Factor–alpha (TNF-alpha):** A cytokine involved in systemic inflammation; elevated levels are often seen in autoimmune diseases and metabolic disorders.
- **Erythrocyte Sedimentation Rate (ESR):** Measures the rate at which red blood cells (erythrocytes) settle; a faster rate suggests the presence of inflammation.
- **Glycosylated Acute-Phase Proteins (GlycA):** This unique marker is often linked to chronic inflammatory states.
- **Interleukin-6 (IL-6):** A pro-inflammatory cytokine involved in the body's immune response and metabolic regulation.

Elevated levels are associated with chronic inflammation and disease progression.

AA/EPA Ratio: This measures the levels of arachidonic acid (an omega-6 fatty acid) relative to eicosapentaenoic acid (an omega-3 fatty acid) in the body. As an indicator of balance between pro-inflammatory and anti-inflammatory processes, a lower ratio is considered healthier. A ratio below 1.5:1 is generally regarded as optimal, though some experts suggest that a range of 1.5 to 3 indicates low risk.

Tests for Environmental Toxins: An Overview

Environmental toxin testing is used to detect the presence of harmful substances that we may be exposed to through air, water, food, or other sources. Over time, chemicals, heavy metals, and pollutants can accumulate in the body, potentially opening the door to chronic health issues. Environmental toxin testing helps assess the risk and impact of toxic exposure, allowing for targeted interventions to reduce or eliminate harmful substances from the body. Here are some of the key tests I look to for this purpose:

Heavy Metal Testing: These tests measure levels of metals such as lead, mercury, aluminum, arsenic, and cadmium in the blood, urine, or hair. High levels can cause various health problems, including neurological and organ damage.

Volatile Organic Compounds (VOC) Testing: VOCs, found in products such as paints, solvents, and cleaning agents, can be tested via blood or urine samples. Exposure to VOCs is linked to respiratory issues, headaches, and long-term risks like cancer.

Pesticide Testing: Blood or urine tests can detect residues of pesticides, herbicides, and insecticides, which are common in food and the environment. Chronic exposure is associated with disruptions of the neurological, reproductive, and endocrine systems.

Phthalates and Bisphenol A (BPA) Testing: These chemicals, commonly found in plastics, can be measured in urine. High levels have been linked to hormonal imbalances, infertility issues, and developmental problems.

Mycotoxin Testing: These tests measure mold toxins, which can accumulate in the body from exposure to mold-contaminated environments. Mycotoxins can cause a range of symptoms, including respiratory issues, fatigue, and immune dysfunction.

A Few Allergy and Immune Function Tests: Hair, Saliva, and Blood

Allergy Testing

Blood Tests (IgE): Blood tests measure immunoglobulin E (IgE) to detect specific allergies such as food, pollen, and pet dander. A high IgE announces an allergic reaction.

Saliva Tests: Less commonly used for allergies, saliva tests can sometimes assess stress hormones (such as cortisol) affecting immune responses.

Hair Tests: Some alternative labs claim to detect sensitivities via hair, but such tests are not widely accepted in mainstream medicine.

Immune Function Testing

Blood Tests: The most reliable include a complete blood count (CBC) for white blood cell counts and T cell/B cell function tests to evaluate immune health. Cytokine profiles offer insights into inflammation or autoimmune conditions.

Saliva Tests: Often used to measure cortisol and secretory immunoglobulin-A (IgA), key indicators of stress and immune health, particularly in mucosal immunity.

> **Hair Tests:** Rarely used for immune function and considered unreliable in conventional medicine, although some alternative practices use them to check for mineral imbalances.

As we've explored, personalized testing in VitalLife provides the foundation for understanding your unique biological makeup and how your body is aging. Armed with this knowledge, we can take targeted action to address imbalances, optimize health, and slow the aging process. But the insights gained from biomarkers, genetic testing, and metabolic assessments are just the beginning—they allow us to pinpoint exactly where interventions are needed to enhance your vitality and longevity.

What lies ahead is truly remarkable: a journey into the frontier of regenerative and longevity medicine where cutting-edge science meets time-tested healing traditions. So, let's start this journey with the fascinating, and at times secretive, world of regenerative treatments.

CHAPTER 8

Unleashing the Power of Regenerative Medicine: Turning Back the Clock

> Hope lies in dreams, in imagination, and in the courage of those who wish to make those dreams a reality.
> —Dr. Jonas Salk, American virologist responsible for developing the polio vaccine (1914–1995)

> I think that in the twenty-first century, medical biology will advance at a more rapid pace than before.
> —Dr. Shinya Yamanaka, Japanese stem cell researcher and Nobel Prize laureate (born 1962)

Now let us unlock the secrets of regenerative and anti-aging medicine, where the power to heal, rejuvenate, and turn back the clock is no longer science fiction but a reality within our reach. Imagine being able to reverse the biological clock and regain the vitality of your younger self—that's exactly what Bryan Johnson, a forty-six-year-old billionaire entrepreneur, is pursuing through his Project Blueprint. Johnson has embraced the potential of regenerative medicine, aiming not only to extend his lifespan but also to enhance his healthspan—the years lived in peak physical and mental health. Over the past few years, he has invested millions in a highly structured regimen, combining stem cell therapies, personalized healthcare, and a rigorous lifestyle to rejuvenate his body from the inside out. It is also reported that he subjects himself to a vast array of tests and experiments, including total plasma exchanges, his son's blood plasma transfusions (parabiosis), microneedling, full-body LED exposure, and MRI scans, to name a few.

One of the more remarkable aspects of Johnson's approach is the use of stem cells, including infusion of stem cells and treatments aimed at repairing his joints, muscles, and even internal organs. It was reported in the media that Johnson recently traveled to the Bahamas to undergo a treatment involving stem cells sourced from young, healthy donors, which were injected into his joints to reduce inflammation, eliminate pain, and enhance mobility. The goal of these stem cell treatments is to restore his body's youthful function by encouraging cellular repair and regeneration.

What sets his protocol apart is not just the use of cutting-edge stem cell treatments, but his comprehensive, data-driven approach to health. His team of more than thirty doctors meticulously monitors every aspect of his physiology, from heart function to lung capacity, and implements treatments designed to reverse aging. As per reports in the media, Johnson's results are noteworthy: his biological age has decreased, with metrics showing the heart of a thirty-seven-year-old, the skin of someone in their late twenties, and improved lung function.

While his methods may seem extreme to some, Johnson's journey is opening up new possibilities in regenerative medicine and anti-aging science. It illustrates the extraordinary potential of harnessing the body's own healing mechanisms through stem cells and personalized therapies. Johnson's work is pushing the boundaries of what's possible in our quest for longevity and youthfulness. His story underscores the transformative power of regenerative medicine for those seeking to turn back the clock on aging.

The Key Principles Behind Regenerative Therapies

Regenerative medicine is revolutionizing modern healthcare and transforming how we approach healing and longevity. Rather than merely treating symptoms or slowing disease progression, regenerative medicine takes a proactive stance, targeting the underlying causes of aging, chronic disease, and degeneration. By harnessing the body's own biological processes, this field offers the potential to repair, restore, and even regenerate damaged tissues, making it possible to dial back conditions once considered irreversible.

The *cornerstone of regenerative medicine is cellular repair and regeneration.* As we age, our body's natural ability to repair damaged tissues weakens, sapping our energy, saddling us with chronic pain, brain fog, and muscle loss—all hallmarks of aging that often result in age-related diseases. Regenerative therapies specifically target these declines, stimulating the body's natural healing mechanisms to rejuvenate tissues and restore function.

The VitalLife program, *refined and updated over the years*, integrates many of these groundbreaking therapies safely and effectively to address a broad range of health concerns—from degenerative diseases and autoimmune conditions to the general effects of aging. This *comprehensive, personalized, and data-driven approach* has helped thousands of patients reclaim their vitality, enhance their performance, and live with greater energy and youthfulness.

By improving tissue health, reducing inflammation, and boosting cellular function, these regenerative treatments help with:

- **Cellular Senescence:** Eliminating or rejuvenating aged cells that promote inflammation to enhance tissue health.
- **Chronic Inflammation:** Regenerative therapies reduce cellular inflammation, a driver of many age-related diseases.

- **Mitochondrial Dysfunction:** Restoring mitochondrial health improves energy and vitality.
- **Metabolic Insulin Resistance:** Enhancing insulin sensitivity reduces inflammation and reverses age-related metabolic decline.

Regenerative Medicine's Impact on Diseases

The applications of regenerative medicine in *anti-aging, orthopedics, cardiovascular health, cosmetic rejuvenation, and chronic disease management* have shown remarkable potential to improve patient outcomes. For example, studies demonstrate that regenerative therapies can significantly reduce the need for major surgeries such as joint replacement. In a 2020 review of clinical trials, patients who received regenerative treatments for knee osteoarthritis reported a 50 percent to 75 percent reduction in pain and significant improvement in mobility compared to those who received traditional therapies.

In cardiovascular health, regenerative medicine has made strides in repairing damaged heart tissue following a heart attack. Patient studies indicate that, in addition to regenerating heart muscle, these treatments can stimulate the regeneration of blood vessels, too, potentially reducing mortality rates and enhancing heart function in patients with ischemic heart disease. These therapies represent a shift from simply managing symptoms to actively repairing tissue and improving long-term heart health.

In VitalLife, I've taken these scientific advancements and translated them into tangible, real-world results for my patients. By integrating regenerative therapies with biomarker testing, genetic analysis, and lifestyle interventions, I design an ultra-personalized treatment plan tailored to each person's unique needs. Regenerative medicine in my practice is not only about managing existing conditions but also about preventing diseases before they develop.

> Regenerative therapies in VitalLife target cellular regeneration, inflammation, cell dysfunction, and insulin resistance.

As we explore these groundbreaking treatments, imagine a future where conditions like arthritis, heart disease, or cognitive decline are not only treatable but also potentially reversible. Regenerative medicine offers us the tools to slow, or even halt, the physical effects of aging, and it's already transforming lives. These advancements have the potential to extend lifespan and significantly enhance the quality of life. While early adopters may be those with wealth and access, regenerative medicine's future is for everyone. No longer confined to elite health resorts, this field is becoming a reality, and we're only beginning to tap into its potential.

Let me add this here: *although I have been using many of the treatments discussed in this book, not all are part of my practice.* Some options, particularly intravenous infusions of cellular and acellular (containing cellular components but not cells, such as exosomes) products, are unavailable in the United States due to restrictions from the Food and Drug Administration (FDA), the government agency tasked with regulating and ensuring the safety of food, drugs, cosmetics, and other products. As a result, individuals seeking these cutting-edge therapies often travel abroad to countries like Switzerland, Germany, and Costa Rica. However, I strongly advise against pursuing such treatments in less-regulated regions of the world such as Mexico, South America, Asia, and the Caribbean. The risks in these areas often outweigh any potential benefits due to inconsistent standards of care and oversight.

Current Regenerative Therapies in Use in the United States and Worldwide

With advances in technology over the past many years, the cost of many regenerative therapies has actually decreased over time. And although the majority of these treatments are not covered by healthcare insurance plans, these treatments are fast becoming affordable options for individuals committed to investing in their long-term health.

Let us now learn in detail about these practical clinical regenerative and anti-aging modalities being used today in the United States and around the globe, although not all are part of VitalLife.

> Many of these regenerative treatments are usually combined in a personalized protocol. Adding other VitalLife modalities to address insulin resistance and inflammation, as discussed in later chapters, provides a comprehensive plan for optimal results.

Therapeutic Plasma Exchange (TPE)

Therapeutic plasma exchange, also called plasmapheresis, removes harmful substances from plasma, the liquid part of the blood, and is traditionally used to treat autoimmune diseases and certain blood disorders. However, it has started to gain attention in clinical practices focused on anti-aging and longevity. In TPE, blood is drawn from the patient, and then separated into plasma (the liquid part of the blood) and the cellular components like red and white blood cells. The plasma, which contains inflammatory markers, metabolic waste, and aging-related proteins, is either filtered or replaced with fresh plasma or a plasma substitute. The blood cells are then mixed with the treated or new plasma and returned to the patient.

In practice, TPE for anti-aging and longevity is still experimental, but some wellness centers, especially in Europe and also at luxury resorts here in the United States, offer it in combination with other therapies aimed at optimizing health, such as exosome and stem cell infusions, hormone replacement, nutritional support, and other IV infusions. Patients who undergo TPE for anti-aging purposes typically report enhanced energy, skin appearance, mental clarity, and overall well-being. Some claim that it helps them feel rejuvenated, with greater vitality and muscle strength.

TPE must be conducted under strict medical supervision, as it involves manipulating blood components and can affect your electrolyte balance, blood volume, and overall circulation. Patients are monitored carefully during and after the procedure to ensure safety and to manage any potential side effects, such as low blood pressure or dizziness. Most sessions last between one and two hours, and multiple sessions may be required over a period of weeks or months, depending on individual goals and health conditions.

Potential Anti-aging Effects

TPE works by removing inflammatory markers and other aging-related molecules from the plasma to create a healthier, less inflammatory environment in the body. The theory is that this process helps to:

- **Reduce Inflammation:** Systemic and chronic low-grade inflammation, common with aging, are linked to many age-related diseases. By removing inflammatory substances from the plasma, plasmapheresis may help reduce overall inflammation in the body.
- **Improve Cellular Health:** The removal of metabolic waste and harmful proteins from plasma is thought to improve the health and function of cells, potentially slowing down cellular aging.
- **Enhance Tissue Regeneration:** With reduced inflammation and improved cellular function, the body's natural ability to repair tissues and heal may be enhanced, contributing to a more youthful appearance and improved physical health.

TPE or plasmapheresis is being explored in the clinical setting as a promising tool for those seeking longevity, and youthfulness.

While more research is needed to fully validate its effectiveness for these purposes, its ability to cleanse the blood of aging-related factors has sparked hope for improved long-term health and vitality.

Senolytics: Removing the Zombie Cells

In my clinical practice, I've seen the incredible impact senolytics can have in combating cellular aging. These compounds target senescent cells, aka the zombie cells we talked about in earlier chapters—the old, dysfunctional cells that build up in the body, fueling inflammation and age-related conditions like arthritis, cardiovascular disease, and cognitive decline. In VitalLife, I've integrated powerful senolytic compounds into personalized treatments, harnessing their ability to promote cellular regeneration and enhance overall health. By clearing out these damaged cells, we not only reduce inflammation but also create an environment where healthier, younger cells can thrive.

One of my cornerstone senolytics is *fisetin*, found in strawberries and apples. Studies show that this natural flavonoid can selectively eliminate senescent cells while sparing healthy ones, reducing chronic inflammation and extending lifespan. Fisetin also bolsters the body's antioxidant defenses, fighting oxidative stress to support cellular health. Alongside fisetin, I also use *quercetin*, another powerful flavonoid that, when combined with a third candidate, *dasatinib*, shows impressive effects on joint health and inflammation, particularly in individuals with osteoarthritis. Together these compounds enhance physical function, reduce pain, and improve mobility.

In addition to these, I incorporate *pterostilbene*, a compound similar to resveratrol, known for its senolytic benefits and its support of mitochondrial function—crucial for sustaining energy and metabolic health as we age. Pterostilbene combats age-related decline by reducing oxidative stress and promoting cellular repair.

Rhodiola, an adaptogenic cold-climate herb with a long history of use in traditional medicine, particularly in Russia, Scandinavia, and other parts of Europe, also plays an important role in countering stress-induced cellular aging. By fortifying the body's resilience against physical and emotional stress, rhodiola helps delay cell senescence and supports faster regeneration. Another unique addition to my senolytic regimen is *chestnut rose*, celebrated in Chinese medicine for its anti-inflammatory properties. High in vitamin C, it promotes collagen production and tissue repair, making it especially valuable for skin elasticity and overall cellular health.

Rapamycin, a groundbreaking senolytic, inhibits the mTOR signaling pathway—a complex cellular network crucial for regulating cell growth, metabolism, and autophagy—playing a pivotal role in slowing cellular aging. Research on rapamycin highlights its potential to extend longevity by clearing senescent cells and reducing cellular stress. It's a key part of my tool kit, and we will discuss it in greater length in chapter 14 on compounded personalized medicines.

These senolytics work in synergy with other regenerative therapies to drive deep cellular rejuvenation. Patients report enhanced energy, mental clarity, and physical function, along with a slower pace of biological aging. This holistic, evidence-based approach not only adds years to life—it also enhances healthspan.

Senolytics represent a significant advancement in regenerative medicine, delivering measurable improvements in biomarkers and lowering the risks of age-related diseases. With ongoing research and clinical trials, the potential of these compounds continues to grow, and I'm proud to offer these advanced treatments to my patients.

Young Blood Transfusions: Parabiosis for Anti-aging and Youthfulness

Now let's talk about parabiosis, a procedure that has stirred up a good deal of controversy even among longevity and regenerative experts. Although studies involving animals have revealed a limited anti-aging effect, *I do not currently recommend or offer parabiosis*, as more data are needed regarding its effectiveness.

Parabiosis is an experimental procedure that involves the joining of the circulatory systems of two organisms. It typically involves connecting the bloodstream of an older organism with that of a younger one. The idea behind this practice is that the younger blood may provide rejuvenating factors to help the older organism's stem cells to regain a better regenerative capacity, potentially reversing some aspects of aging and promoting youthfulness.

The concept of parabiosis builds on the pioneering work of Sir John Gurdon, the Nobel Prize–winning British biologist who demonstrated that adult cells have the remarkable capacity to regenerate when placed in a younger, healthier environment. His findings revealed that adult cells could adapt and differentiate as if they were native embryonic cells, showcasing their potential for rejuvenation.

The interest in parabiosis as an anti-aging therapy emerged from animal studies, particularly in mice, where researchers found that older mice, when connected to younger mice, showed improvements in various markers of aging. For example, the older mice experienced enhanced tissue repair, improved cognitive function, and increased muscle regeneration. This led to speculation that factors in young blood—such as certain proteins, growth factors, and other molecules—might help restore vitality and slow the aging process in older individuals.

The primary mechanism involves reducing chronic inflammation, which is a key driver of aging. This is achieved by decreasing the levels of pro-inflammatory cytokines in aged tissues, thus enhancing overall tissue health and cellular repair. Moreover, parabiosis has been shown to boost mitochondrial function, which helps improve the cell's ability to produce energy efficiently and reduces oxidative stress—a major contributor to cellular damage and aging. Additionally, in the brain, it promotes *neurogenesis* (generation and development of new functional neurons in the adult brain) and supports cognitive function by activating neural stem cells, particularly in regions like the *hippocampus*, which are crucial for memory and learning.

On a biological level, *parabiosis has demonstrated positive effects on key biomarkers associated with aging*, such as inflammation markers, mitochondrial efficiency, and overall metabolic health. This suggests that parabiosis holds potential not just for extending lifespan, but for improving healthspan, offering significant benefits across multiple organ systems.

More rigorous scientific investigation is needed before it can be considered a safe and effective treatment.

Ozone Therapy for Anti-aging and Youthfulness

Ozone therapy can be a powerful, innovative treatment for many. It is quickly gaining recognition for its potential in anti-aging and rejuvenation. Ozone (O_3) is a highly reactive form of oxygen that, when introduced into the body in precise amounts, activates a wide range of healing and regenerative processes.

A core benefit of ozone therapy is its ability to improve oxygen delivery to tissues. As we age, our cells become less efficient at using oxygen, leading to oxidative stress, inflammation, and cellular damage. Ozone therapy addresses this by *boosting oxygen utilization and circulation*, which helps cells repair and regenerate more effectively. This increased oxygen availability supports detoxification, reduces inflammation, and stimulates the production of antioxidant enzymes that protect cells from further damage.

Ozone therapy is also shown to enhance the immune system, activating the body's natural healing mechanisms. It helps modulate immune responses and reduce chronic inflammation. In addition, by improving mitochondrial function—the cell's energy centers—ozone therapy boosts energy levels, metabolism, and overall vitality.

For those seeking a more youthful appearance, ozone therapy can reduce fatigue, improve skin elasticity, and promote a radiant, refreshed look. Its ability to rejuvenate tissues and stimulate collagen production makes it a highly appealing option for skin health and anti-aging.

Though still considered unconventional in some circles, the growing popularity of ozone therapy reflects its potential to support healthy aging and enhance quality of life. Regular ozone treatments can help slow the aging process, increase energy levels, and equip the body with the tools it needs to stay youthful and vibrant longer.

Hyperbaric Oxygen Therapy for Anti-aging and Youthfulness

Hyperbaric oxygen therapy (HBOT) is a cutting-edge treatment that is increasingly being used to combat the effects of aging and promote youthfulness. It has become a popular tool among professional athletes and celebrities for enhancing recovery, performance, and beauty. Many rich and famous people are buying these chambers for their personal use in their homes. In HBOT, individuals breathe pure oxygen in a pressurized chamber, which *boosts oxygen delivery to tissues*. This helps reduce inflammation and speed healing and recovery from injuries—a major advantage for athletes in sports such as football and basketball.

I have found that one of the key regenerative and anti-aging benefits of HBOT is its *ability to stimulate the production of new stem cells*, which play a vital role in tissue repair and regeneration. As we age, our stem cell activity declines, leading to slower healing and reduced tissue renewal. HBOT helps activate dormant stem cells, encouraging the body to repair damaged tissues, enhance skin elasticity, and promote a more youthful appearance. The increased oxygen also boosts collagen production, which can reduce wrinkles and improve skin texture.

Moreover, HBOT significantly improves mitochondrial function—the energy factories of our cells. By enhancing oxygen delivery, the therapy supports better energy production, which leads to increased vitality, sharper mental clarity, and improved physical performance. HBOT also reduces inflammation, another hallmark of aging, by stimulating the body's natural anti-inflammatory processes. This reduction in chronic inflammation not only supports skin health but also helps protect against age-related diseases such as cardiovascular disease and cognitive decline.

Studies have shown that HBOT can even lengthen telomeres—the protective caps on the ends of chromosomes that shorten as we age. Shortened telomeres are associated with cellular aging and increased disease risk. By promoting telomere lengthening, HBOT offers a unique way to counteract one of the fundamental biological processes of aging.

In my experience, hyperbaric oxygen therapy (HBOT) offers significant benefits beyond sports injuries and skin rejuvenation. I've found it especially helpful for conditions such as long COVID, concussions, dementia, chronic fatigue syndrome, chronic wounds, fibromyalgia, and Lyme disease. Typically, I recommend a series of sessions lasting sixty to ninety minutes each, *integrating HBOT into a comprehensive plan alongside other advanced treatments*, such as stem cell and exosome therapies and cosmetic laser rejuvenation. This combined approach helps patients achieve optimal healing and revitalization.

While hyperbaric oxygen therapy (HBOT) is generally safe and well tolerated, I do advise patients that, like any treatment, it can have side effects, and it's essential to monitor for certain reactions. Common side effects include mild ear discomfort or sinus pressure due to the pressurization process, similar to the sensation experienced during air travel. Occasionally, patients may experience temporary vision changes, which typically resolve after treatment. Some individuals may also feel lightheaded or fatigued following a session, but these effects are usually short-lived.

In rare cases, prolonged or high-pressure HBOT can lead to oxygen toxicity, which may adversely affect the lungs or central nervous system. To ensure safety, it's important to work with a trained professional who can adjust treatment protocols based on your individual health needs, especially for those with conditions such as chronic sinus issues, claustrophobia, and a history of lung disease. By carefully monitoring each session and adjusting treatment as needed, patients can safely benefit from the rejuvenating effects of HBOT.

HBOT offers a powerful, noninvasive approach to anti-aging. Whether it's improving skin health, boosting energy, or supporting cognitive function, HBOT has the potential to help you feel and look younger, longer.

Medical Technologies in Use for Anti-aging and Vitality

In the quest for anti-aging and vitality, cutting-edge technological devices are becoming essential in personalized health and wellness strategies. While many of these advanced devices are available in wellness clinics, an increasing number of the wealthy individuals are investing hundreds of thousands of dollars to bring them into their homes. This private access allows them to use the latest noninvasive technologies regularly, integrating them into daily routines to combat aging, stimulate cellular regeneration, and promote healing.

Infrared and Near-Infrared Therapy

Infrared (IR, with wavelengths of 900+ nm) and near-infrared (NIR, with wavelengths of 810-850 nm) therapy penetrate the skin to stimulate cells and tissues at deeper levels. These wavelengths of light heat tissues below the skin's surface, which helps increase circulation, promote collagen production, and aid in tissue repair. This has made infrared therapy particularly popular in skin rejuvenation and anti-aging aesthetic practices, as it can help reduce the appearance of wrinkles and improve skin elasticity. The increased circulation also promotes muscle recovery, making it useful for athletes and individuals who prioritize physical health and youthful performance.

Infrared and NIR light stimulate mitochondrial activity, helping cells produce more energy (ATP) and reducing oxidative stress, which are critical factors in maintaining vitality and slowing the aging process. It can improve energy, cognitive functioning, and physical performance with regular sessions.

LED Light Therapy

LED light therapy is another popular technological device in the realm of anti-aging. It uses various wavelengths of light-emitting diodes (LED) to target skin cells. Different colors of LED light—for instance, red and blue—offer distinct benefits. Red light therapy (with wavelengths of 630-660 nm) penetrates deep into the skin and is known for boosting collagen production, reducing fine lines, and improving overall skin tone and texture. Blue light therapy (with wavelengths of 400-470 nm), on the other hand, is used for treating acne and reducing inflammation. Over time, regular use of LED light therapy can improve the appearance of aging skin and promote a more youthful, radiant complexion.

Pulsed Electromagnetic Field Therapy (PEMF)

PEMF therapy uses electromagnetic fields to stimulate cellular function and repair tissues. The therapy is based on the principle that electromagnetic fields can interact with the body's natural electrical currents, enhancing cell regeneration, reducing pain, and improving overall energy levels. PEMF devices are commonly used to treat chronic pain, accelerate bone healing, and promote general wellness. When applied for anti-aging, PEMF therapy may improve circulation, reduce inflammation, and enhance cellular repair—helping users feel more energetic and youthful.

Cryotherapy

It's another technological device widely used for anti-aging. By exposing the body to extreme cold temperatures for short durations, cryotherapy triggers vasoconstriction (narrowing of blood vessels) and endorphin release, which can reduce inflammation, numb pain, and promote recovery; it also reduces wrinkles and improves skin tone. It's often used for pain management, reducing swelling, aiding muscle recovery, and even improving skin conditions. Some studies suggest potential benefits for neurodegenerative conditions, though further research is needed. It is also popular among professional athletes for recovery and inflammation management and is also gaining traction in the anti-aging field for its ability to promote collagen production and rejuvenate the skin.

Electrical Muscle Stimulation (EMS)

Electrical Muscle Stimulation (EMS) is a technology used to enhance muscle contraction by sending electrical impulses to muscles, causing them to contract involuntarily. EMS is often used in physical therapy to aid in muscle recovery and strengthen weakened muscles. However, it is also gaining popularity as a fitness and anti-aging tool to help tone muscles, improve circulation, and maintain muscle mass, which tends to decline with age. Regular use can lead to improved strength, toned muscles, and better overall physical performance—helping individuals retain a more youthful appearance and function.

—

For those seeking to extend their healthspan and maintain youthful vitality, integrating these devices into a personalized wellness plan offers a cutting-edge approach to staying at their peak for longer.

As we conclude our exploration of regenerative medicine treatments currently in use around the globe, many of which are incorporated within VitalLife, it's evident that these therapies are transforming how we address aging and wellness. *Many of these are usually combined together in a personalized protocol. Also, adding other modalities to address insulin resistance and inflammation provides a comprehensive plan for optimal results.*

With this solid foundation of regenerative techniques, we now turn to the remarkable potential of stem cell and exosome therapies. In the next chapter, we'll delve into how these advanced treatments tap into the body's innate regenerative power to support lasting vitality and youthful energy.

CHAPTER 9

Stem Cells and Exosomes: Stimulating Cellular Regeneration

> Stem cell research is the key to developing cures for degenerative conditions like Parkinson's and motor neuron disease, from which I and many others suffer.
> —Sir Stephen Hawking, British theoretical physicist and cosmologist (1942–2018)

> Without a doubt, stem cell research will lead to the dramatic improvement in the human condition and will benefit millions of people.
> —Eli Broad, American businessman and philanthropist (1933–2021)

For over twenty years, I've been honored to practice specialized treatments that transform lives. As the field has evolved, I've continuously updated protocols at VitalLife to stay at the forefront of the latest clinical advancements. Today, I'm excited to share how regenerative medicine—using stem cells and exosomes—is reshaping our understanding of health and healing in truly groundbreaking ways. Imagine the extraordinary possibility of repairing, regenerating, and rejuvenating your body from the inside out—this is the groundbreaking promise of regenerative treatments like stem cells and exosomes.

I am sure many of you have noticed that stem cell therapies have gained remarkable popularity over the past few years, capturing the attention of medical professionals, researchers, and the public alike. Once limited to research labs, stem cell treatments are now being applied in clinics worldwide to address a variety of conditions, from joint pain and sports injuries to neurodegenerative diseases and chronic conditions such as diabetes and lupus.

The media coverage of high-profile athletes and well-known individuals using these therapies has further propelled their prominence, creating widespread awareness and curiosity. Prominent professional athletes and prominent figures, including Tiger Woods, Cristiano Ronaldo, Rafael Nadal, Jack Nicklaus, Peyton Manning, the late Kobe Bryant, Steph Curry, and Tony Robbins have been reported in the media to have utilized stem cell treatments. Many of these high-profile individuals sought these therapies outside the United States.

I have mentioned earlier that, over the years, I've worked with patients who had to travel to medical centers in Switzerland, Germany, and Costa Rica to access these therapies. However, I continue to advise everybody against pursuing these treatments in less regulated regions such as Mexico, South America, Asia, or the Caribbean. The risks in these areas often outweigh the potential benefits due to inconsistent standards of care and oversight.

> For the best possible results, the VitalLife program utilizes a comprehensive and integrated approach with regenerative therapies, designing a customized protocol that includes several regenerative therapies combined with lifestyle, metabolic, and anti-inflammation strategies.

By tailoring each plan to an individual's unique medical needs and goals, I develop a *personalized protocol that integrates many of the regenerative and other therapies* discussed in this book. For example, a patient with joint degeneration may benefit from a series of **PRP** injections for immediate inflammation relief and from stem cell therapy for longer-term tissue regeneration. Similarly, for aesthetic goals, combining exosomes with **PRP** and laser facial rejuvenation enhances collagen production and improves skin texture, delivering not only surface-level improvements but deeper, lasting changes.

These regenerative therapies can also be integrated with broader components of this program, including hormone optimization, hyperbaric oxygen therapy, IV infusions, personalized pharmacy products, and anti-inflammatory protocols. This integration of regenerative treatments with other targeted modalities ensures that all aspects of health are addressed—maximizing the benefits and supporting sustainable, long-term results. This *multifaceted approach* aligns each treatment element to work harmoniously, delivering the best possible outcomes for health, vitality, and longevity.

While the potential benefits are impressive, it's essential to approach these therapies with caution. They come with risks, costs, and limited knowledge of long-term outcomes. With proper review of medical issues and patients' biology, the risks can be minimized or even completely avoided.

So, What Exactly Are These Stem Cells and Exosomes?

Now, let me introduce you to cellular bioactive products, which involve using whole cells such as stem cells, and acellular bioactive products, which utilize only specific components of cells such as exosomes. Stem cells are unique cells within the body that have two defining abilities: *self-renewal* (the capacity to divide and produce more cells) and *differentiation* (the ability to transform into specialized cells, such as muscle, bone, or nerve cells). These cells are crucial in both development and tissue repair, as they serve as the body's natural repair system.

Allogeneic stem cells come from a donor, typically someone younger and healthier, which makes them highly effective for regenerative therapies, due to their stronger ability to promote tissue repair, reduce inflammation, and support immune function. These cells are particularly useful for systemic treatments to tackle anti-aging or chronic disease management.

In contrast, *autologous stem cells* are harvested from a person's own body, usually from bone marrow or fat tissue. While autologous cells have reduced risk of immune rejection—where the body's defenses attack the donor cells as trespassers—their effectiveness diminishes with age, as older cells lose their regenerative potential. While autologous cells can be effective for localized therapies, allogeneic stem cells generally offer broader, more potent benefits in regenerative medicine.

Based on their origin, there are several types of stem cells used in regenerative medicine, each with unique properties and capabilities. Understanding the differences between these types is key to knowing how they can be applied to various treatments, whether for anti-aging, disease management, or tissue regeneration.

Embryonic Stem Cells (ESCs): These are *pluripotent* stem cells, which means they have the ability to develop into any type of cell in the body. Derived from early-stage embryos, ESCs are highly versatile and have immense potential for regenerating damaged tissues or organs. However, their use is controversial due to ethical concerns surrounding the source of these cells, and their application is restricted in many parts of the world, including the United States. Currently embryonic stem cells are used in scientific laboratories for research and clinical trials under FDA supervision, especially for eye conditions such as age-related macular degeneration and retinitis pigmentosa, and cardiovascular illnesses such as heart attack and chronic heart failure.

Adult Stem Cells (ASCs): These are *multipotent* stem cells found in various tissues throughout the body, such as bone marrow, fat (adipose tissue), and blood. While not as versatile as embryonic stem cells, they are still capable of differentiating into a limited range of cell types, usually related to their tissue of origin. The most commonly used adult stem cells are *hematopoietic* stem cells from bone marrow, which can regenerate blood cells, and *mesenchymal* stem cells (MSCs), typically harvested from bone marrow or fat tissue, which can regenerate bone, cartilage, and muscle. Because adult stem cells are often collected from a person's own body (autologous), they avoid ethical concerns in addition to reducing the risk of being rejected by the immune system.

Induced Pluripotent Stem Cells (iPSCs): The discovery of these types of cells by Japanese scientist Dr. Shinya Yamanaka and his team at the Nara Institute of Science and Technology in 2006 was a major breakthrough in stem cell research, earning him a Nobel Prize. iPSCs are adult cells that have been genetically reprogrammed in the lab to behave like embryonic stem cells. By introducing specific reprogramming factors, scientists can turn a regular skin or blood cell into a pluripotent stem cell capable of becoming any type of cell in the body. iPSCs offer great potential because they combine the versatility of embryonic stem cells with the ethical advantage of being derived from adult tissues. However, iPSC technology is still relatively new, and more research is needed to understand its full potential and any long-term risks.

Perinatal Stem Cells: These stem cells come from perinatal tissues, such as umbilical cord blood and tissue, the placenta, and amniotic fluid. They are typically multipotent, meaning they can differentiate into a variety of cell types, though they are not as versatile as embryonic stem cells. Umbilical cord blood stem cells, for example, are rich in hematopoietic stem cells, which are used in the treatment of blood disorders. These cells are considered immunologically safe and are rejected less often. Because perinatal cells are harvested from tissues that are normally discarded after birth, their use is less controversial ethically.

Each type of stem cell has unique advantages, with the choice depending on the patient's specific needs and the condition being treated. However, regenerative treatments are not limited to stem cells. Let's explore the latest, and potentially superior, advancements in cellular rejuvenation technology.

Exosomes and Extracellular Vesicles (EVs): These acellular couriers come in different sizes and types, with exosomes being smaller in size and one of the well-studied types. Derived from sources such as umbilical cord blood, placental tissue, and bone marrow and fat mesenchymal stem cells, exosomes carry valuable molecular information that can influence the behavior of recipient cells. Unlike stem cell therapy, which involves transplanting whole cells, exosome therapy focuses on using these to trigger the body's natural repair processes without the risk of immune rejection.

Exosomes are now increasingly being used in regenerative medicine. *One of the key advantages of exosome treatments is that they do not contain DNA material*, which significantly enhances their safety profile. Without genetic material, there's a *reduced risk of immune rejection or complications*, making exosomes a highly versatile and safe tool for therapeutic purposes.

As research continues, these therapies could transform the treatment landscape for a wide variety of conditions, promoting healing from within by leveraging the body's natural communication and repair systems.

Intravenous (IV) Infusions of Regenerative Stem Cells and Exosomes

I do not use or recommend intravenous infusions of autologous (your own) stem cells, and here's why. In my view, infusing autologous cells is ineffective and can give people false hope. Physicians should refrain from offering this practice until we have stronger scientific data to support its effectiveness.

While autologous stem cell infusions from a patient's own body are considered safer due to the lower risk of immune rejection, they have limitations that significantly reduce their efficacy in regenerative and anti-aging treatments. One primary concern is that stem cell quality declines with age. Our stem cells incur damage and lose regenerative potential over time, meaning autologous cells taken from an older patient often lack the capacity for effective tissue repair and regeneration compared with those from younger sources, like placental or umbilical cord stem cells. In essence, older stem cells may lack the ability to provide the level of repair required for meaningful progress in treating chronic diseases or achieving anti-aging objectives. Moreover, harvesting these cells from a patient's bone marrow or adipose tissue can also be invasive and uncomfortable, adding further challenges without guaranteeing better outcomes.

In contrast, placental or umbilical stem cell infusions, which are younger and more potent, tend to produce more reliable results in regenerative therapies. These cells are at their peak regenerative potential, with a greater ability to modulate immune responses, reduce inflammation, and promote healing across different tissues. For individuals seeking therapies to support longevity, enhance youthfulness, or manage complex conditions such as autoimmune diseases, placental-derived stem cells present a more effective and viable option.

Exosome infusions, a growing tool in regenerative medicine, are typically derived from the blood and placental tissues of young, healthy individuals—not from embryonic tissues. As I mentioned earlier, one of the primary advantages of exosome treatments, especially in intravenous infusions, is their enhanced safety profile. Because *exosomes contain no DNA material*, there is a reduced risk of immune rejection or complications, making them a versatile and safe therapeutic option.

Intravenous (IV) Placental Stem Cell Infusions for Longevity and Healthspan

Intravenous placental stem cell infusions, available primarily outside the United States, are at the cutting edge of regenerative medicine. The cells are sourced from donated placental tissues after a healthy birth and are rich in mesenchymal stem cells (MSCs), which are known for their regenerative properties. When administered intravenously, placental stem cells can:

- **Reduce Systemic Inflammation:** Chronic inflammation is one of the key contributors to aging, and MSCs are known for their powerful anti-inflammatory properties. These stem cells modulate immune responses, helping to reduce inflammation throughout the body, which in turn helps to slow down age-related diseases such as cardiovascular issues, diabetes, and neurodegeneration.
- **Promote Tissue Repair:** Because placental stem cells have the ability to support tissue regeneration, these enhance the body's natural capacity to heal. This can lead to improvements in organ function, muscle regeneration, and even skin health, providing a more youthful appearance and better overall vitality.
- **Improve Metabolic Function:** These cells can help improve insulin sensitivity and regulate blood sugar levels, which is essential for managing metabolic diseases like type 2 diabetes. By promoting better mitochondrial function

and cellular repair, placental stem cells can address the metabolic imbalances that contribute to aging.
- **Boost Immune Health:** Placental stem cells play a key role in immune modulation, helping the body fight infections more efficiently while preventing the overactive immune responses seen in autoimmune diseases. By rebalancing the immune system, these cells help mitigate disease progression while promoting general health and vitality.

In summary, for those seeking to enhance longevity and healthspan, placental stem cell infusions may provide a means to rejuvenate the body at a cellular level. By reducing inflammation, promoting tissue repair, and balancing the immune system, these therapies address key mechanisms of aging, helping people maintain youthful energy, mental clarity, and overall health. For these treatments, patients usually have to travel to medical clinics outside the United States.

Intravenous Exosome Infusions for Health and Longevity

In addition to stem cells, exosomes derived from placental tissues are also gaining attention for their role in enhancing youthfulness and slowing the signs of aging. Their ability to stimulate tissue repair and regeneration makes intravenous exosome infusions an effective solution for improving cellular function across the body, treating degenerative, metabolic, and autoimmune conditions, and enhancing overall health and performance.

When physicians utilize carefully sourced and safe exosomes, patients often experience notable improvements in tissue regeneration, disease management, and overall health restoration without the risks associated with more invasive therapies. These exosome

IV infusions, available primarily outside the United States, help to do the following:

- **Stimulate Skin Rejuvenation:** Exosomes encourage collagen production, improve skin elasticity, and reduce fine lines and wrinkles, giving the skin a more youthful appearance.
- **Improve Cognitive Function:** Exosomes have also been shown to promote neuroprotection and stimulate the repair of damaged nerve cells, or neurons. By their ability to cross the blood-brain barrier (a protective layer of cells and tissue that surrounds the brain's blood vessels), they can enhance brain function, sharpen memory, and support cognitive health—key elements in maintaining youthfulness. They have also shown promise in neurodegenerative conditions such as Alzheimer's disease, Parkinson's disease, and even in traumatic brain injuries.
- **Boost Energy Levels:** Exosomes, by improving mitochondrial function and reducing cellular damage, enhance energy production at the cellular level, helping individuals experience increased vitality and stamina.
- **Muscle Regeneration:** Exosomes promote muscle regeneration, potentially improving muscle function and mitigating the effects of sarcopenia, a serious age-related muscle loss.
- **Cardiovascular Health:** Exosomes can improve vascularization and new blood vessel formation known as *angiogenesis*, which can help with atherosclerosis, heart disease, and heart failure.
- **Metabolic Health:** Exosomes are also showing promise in helping with insulin resistance, lipid metabolism, and diabetes.

Special Note on Treating Autoimmune and Metabolic Conditions with IV Placental Stem Cells and Exosomes

One of the most exciting applications of placental stem cell infusions and exosomes is in the management of autoimmune and metabolic diseases. For select patients and after due safety protocol, treatments with IV placental cells and exosomes can be good options for several autoimmune and metabolic conditions.

In autoimmune conditions like lupus, multiple sclerosis, rheumatoid arthritis, and chronic fatigue syndrome, the immune system mistakenly attacks the body's own tissues, causing chronic inflammation and tissue damage. In these conditions, placental stem cells and exosomes work to recalibrate the body's defense force, reducing damaging immune responses while promoting tissue repair. This not only helps control symptoms but also slows the progression of the disease.

For metabolic diseases such as insulin resistance and type 2 diabetes, placental stem cells and exosomes can improve metabolic regulation by enhancing insulin sensitivity and promoting healthy cellular metabolism. These therapies have shown promise in reducing blood sugar levels, improving organ function, and decreasing the inflammation that often accompanies metabolic disorders.

Safety and Effectiveness of IV Placental Stem Cells and Exosomes

Placental stem cell and exosome infusions are generally considered safe. Since these are sourced from healthy donors and are processed to remove any DNA material, the risk of rejection or complications is minimal. Placental-derived products offer the advantage of being rich in growth factors and anti-inflammatory proteins, which help accelerate healing and regeneration across the body.

Placental stem cell and exosome infusions represent an exciting frontier in regenerative medicine, providing a holistic approach to longevity, disease management, and youthful vitality. These therapies effectively target inflammation, immune regulation, and cellular repair, offering systemic benefits that enhance healthspan, while addressing chronic conditions like autoimmune and metabolic diseases. As regenerative medicine continues to advance, these infusion therapies are increasingly used worldwide, delivering regenerative effects throughout the body to counteract widespread inflammation, cellular aging, and immune dysfunction. Placental stem cell and exosome infusions hold significant promise for personalized, preventative healthcare, helping individuals sustain health, energy, and well-being for years to come.

Localized, Targeted Stem Cell Procedures

Over the past two decades, I have performed numerous of these localized regenerative procedures in my clinic. These treatments include ultrasound-guided localized injections with platelet-rich plasma (PRP), autologous bone marrow stem cells, and fat-derived stem cells, helping patients recover from a wide range of conditions. These treatments have enabled me to help patients from all over the world in overcoming chronic pain, joint diseases, arthritis, spinal issues, sports injuries, cosmetic concerns, erectile dysfunction, and more.

I began my journey in this field when regenerative medicine was still emerging—a new and evolving specialty practiced by only a handful of physicians in the United States. Drawing on my background in anti-aging and Eastern medicine, I was able to integrate these therapies into a broader, holistic approach. *Very often, I integrate regenerative procedures with other modalities,* such as hormone optimization, customized pharmacy solutions, and lifestyle modifications targeting insulin resistance and chronic inflammation. This comprehensive strategy proved instrumental in achieving exceptional results for my patients—often surpassing outcomes seen in many other practices.

By leveraging your own cells' capacity to heal, we can frequently bypass more invasive options like surgery, offering a powerful alternative that leads to faster recovery and lasting results. I've seen so many patients experience remarkable transformations—from NFL athletes recovering from sports injuries to elderly individuals seeking arthritis improvement, and even celebrities pursuing cosmetic rejuvenation.

> In my experience, after having performed thousands of these procedures over twenty years, the key factors for your best results are selecting patients carefully, using tailored cellular and acellular products with ultrasound guidance (when needed), and utilizing a multifaceted approach that includes several regenerative therapies along with lifestyle, metabolic, and anti-inflammation strategies.

But it is very important to perform these interventions after proper patient selection, thorough testing, and utilizing appropriate customized regenerative products. For safety and optimal results, these procedures also must be incorporated as part of a comprehensive, multifaceted protocol.

Localized Platelet-Rich Plasma (PRP) Therapy

Let's begin with PRP therapy, one of the initial regenerative treatments I started to use in VitalLife. When I first introduced PRP treatments twenty years ago, I was one of the few physicians in the United States utilizing this therapy, and it was largely unknown. Today I see many doctors adopting PRP to support their patients' health, which I consider a positive trend—as long as it is applied individually and integrated into a comprehensive treatment plan.

The procedure itself is straightforward, yet remarkably effective. We start by drawing a small sample of blood, typically from the arm, and placing it in a centrifuge. This process separates the platelet-rich plasma from other blood components, like red and white blood cells. The concentrated PRP solution is then injected directly into the targeted area, be it a painful joint, muscle, tendon, or for cosmetic use.

In my practice, I follow a meticulous PRP preparation process to achieve the highest concentrations of growth factors and bioactive compounds, which I believe are critical for optimal results. Over the years, I've also refined my injection techniques to maximize patient comfort and ensure precise delivery of PRP into the intended areas. Combining PRP with other therapies, such as exosomes, often yields even better outcomes. Conditions that may benefit include the following:

- **Arthritis:** The power of PRP lies in its growth factors, which stimulate the body's natural repair processes, promoting tissue regeneration and reducing inflammation. For patients with conditions like osteoarthritis, PRP injections in the joint can encourage cartilage repair, enhance mobility, and alleviate pain. Many of my patients have regained significant joint mobility after a series of PRP treatments, allowing them to resume activities that were once limited.

- **Sports Medicine:** PRP is also invaluable in sports medicine. Athletes suffering from ligament injuries or tendinitis—common issues that can sideline even elite players—have used PRP to accelerate recovery. The injections help reduce inflammation in damaged ligaments or tendons and speed up healing, often enabling athletes to return to their sport sooner than traditional treatments might allow.
- **Cosmetic Medicine:** PRP facial procedures have gained popularity in nonsurgical esthetics, widely known as the "vampire facial." This technique involves injecting PRP into the skin to stimulate collagen production, reduce fine lines, and improve skin tone and texture. Patients appreciate that it's an entirely natural approach—using their own cells to rejuvenate their skin for a healthier, more youthful look without chemicals or synthetic fillers. These are usually combined with other treatments such as lasers and exosomes.
- **Hair Loss:** For patients dealing with hair loss or thinning, I've also used PRP therapy to promote hair regrowth. While results vary, combining PRP with other treatments, like localized exosome therapy, often enhances the outcome.
- **Erectile Dysfunction (ED):** A series of PRP therapies—also known as *P-shots*—can be transformative for ED. By harnessing the patient's own growth factors and bioactive compounds, PRP injections can significantly improve sexual function and boost confidence. Many of my patients have reported improvements, particularly when the injections are combined with additional modalities such as sound wave therapy (using targeted sound waves to improve blood flow), hormone optimization, and peptide therapy.

Localized Autologous (Your Own) Bone Marrow Stem Cell Treatments

When used properly and following a thorough medical evaluation, I have found bone marrow stem cell treatments to be highly effective in alleviating chronic pain from joint and spinal conditions, promoting healing, and even preventing the need for surgery. Over the years, I have performed these procedures for sports injuries and various musculoskeletal conditions, including chronic arthritis. I adhere to meticulous handling of autologous bone marrow stem cells, strictly following FDA guidelines.

I have had the privilege of helping many professional athletes and high achievers avoid risky surgeries. *This procedure is particularly favored by athletes because it promotes healing without the formation of significant scar tissue*, as scar tissue can limit flexibility and hinder athletic performance. As part of the comprehensive VitalLife program, I always integrate these procedures with other healing modalities, such as personalized post-procedure training protocols, compounded pharmacy products, and tailored supplements.

This nonsurgical outpatient procedure involves extracting stem cells from the patient's own bone marrow, typically from the iliac crest (the back of the hip bone), using a specialized needle in a minimally invasive procedure. Patients remain awake during the extraction, but a local anesthetic renders it relatively painless. After collecting the bone marrow aspirate, we process it to concentrate the mesenchymal stem cells (MSCs), which have the remarkable ability to differentiate into various cell types—such as cartilage, bone, and muscle. The concentrated stem cells are then injected directly into the area of concern, usually under ultrasound guidance, whether that's an arthritic joint or the area around a damaged spinal disc.

While this therapy may not be as effective for advanced or "bone-on-bone" disease, where the protective cartilage on the end of bones has been denuded, many of my patients with mild to moderate osteoarthritis, particularly in the knees or hips, have experienced life-changing results. These injections reduce joint inflammation, provide long-lasting pain relief, and often stimulate cartilage regeneration. Many patients find that bone marrow stem cell therapy helps them regain mobility and avoid joint replacement surgery.

For chronic neck and back pain from soft tissue spine injuries and degenerative disease, bone marrow stem cells can be injected into the ligaments and the damaged *vertebral facet joint* area. The cells work to regenerate tissue, improving both pain, flexibility, and function. I've seen numerous patients, previously told that surgery was their only option, achieve significant improvements with these stem cell therapies, allowing them to live pain-free without invasive surgery.

These autologous bone marrow cells can also be used for other applications, such as ED and facial wrinkle rejuvenation, but with limited results.

Localized Autologous (Your Own) Fat-Derived Stem Cell Treatments

Similar to bone marrow-derived stem cells, I have found that fat-derived stem cells can offer another effective regenerative treatment for many people. This entails harvesting adipose tissue through a (mini) liposuction procedure. The fat is typically taken from areas like the side of the abdominal wall or inner thighs. Once the fat is harvested, it is processed in a laboratory to extract adipose-derived stem cells, which are then reinjected into the targeted area.

What's unique about fat-derived stem cells is their high concentration of mesenchymal stem cells, which are particularly effective at regenerating soft tissue and cartilage. MSC cells are *ideal for treating joint degeneration*, particularly in larger joints like the shoulders, knees, and hips. Patients with chronic pain or injuries to these joints have experienced significant relief and improved function after just a few treatments.

In the field of aesthetics, fat grafting combined with stem cells has been transformative. Patients seeking natural facial rejuvenation or volume restoration prefer this method because it uses their own fat, enriched with stem cells, to plump and restore youthful contours in the face. Unlike synthetic fillers, which may need to be replaced over time, fat-derived stem cells continue to work within the body to promote long-lasting skin regeneration.

As with bone marrow cells, autologous fat cells can also be used for other applications such as ED, but with limited results and a higher risk of side effects than other treatment modalities such as exosomes and PRP.

Special Note: Chronic Joint, Neck, and Low Back Pain

For the past twenty years, I have seen how these therapies have transformed the lives of so many patients with chronic low back and neck pain due to arthritis or soft tissue injuries, often from car accidents or falls. Under ultrasound guidance, PRP and bone marrow–derived stem cells are injected into the soft tissue areas of the spine and vertebral facet joints, where they stimulate tissue repair. This approach is particularly effective for soft tissue injuries, where traditional treatments often provide only temporary relief. Stem cell therapy helps rebuild soft tissue and joint material, reduce inflammation, and alleviate chronic pain—all without the need for invasive surgery.

Similarly, as I mentioned earlier, patients suffering from chronic pain due to arthritis, injuries, or other conditions in their knees, hips, or other major joints have found significant relief. Stem cell and PRP therapies improve joint function, reduce inflammation and pain, and may even support cartilage regeneration, allowing patients to avoid or delay joint replacement surgery.

Special Note: Treatments for Erectile Dysfunction (ED)

A particularly revolutionary application of these cellular and acellular therapies has been in treating erectile dysfunction (ED). It is a common issue, affecting millions of men worldwide, particularly as they age. The primary cause is often arterial blockage, which reduces blood flow—a condition linked to aging, diabetes, high blood pressure, and lifestyle factors. Despite its vast prevalence, it is mostly underreported, as men hesitate to seek treatment for this condition. Yet, it is crucial to address this for both physical and emotional well-being. Effective therapies are now available, offering the chance to restore function, confidence, and quality of life.

For many men, I use a series of PRP injections, known as the P-shot, to rejuvenate the tissue, improve blood flow, and restore function. Sometimes stem cells derived from autologous bone marrow and fat can also be used. The stem cells and P-shot involve injecting directly into local cavernous tissue, where they stimulate the growth of new blood vessels, nerves, and tissues. These offer a natural and noninvasive alternative to dangerous implant surgeries as well as medications such as Viagra and Cialis, especially when these medicines fail to work or cause side effects.

In more advanced cases of ED, *several modalities are combined as a multi-session approach*, offering a more comprehensive regenerative treatment protocol. Some clinics have recently started using exosomes for this purpose as well (discussed below). These therapies not only address the symptoms but also work to repair and rejuvenate the underlying tissues. Many men who have undergone these treatments report dramatic improvements in both their sexual performance and their confidence.

Localized, Targeted Exosome Treatments

As we have discussed, exosomes have emerged as one of the most exciting advancements in regenerative medicine, offering transformative potential in cosmetic rejuvenation, musculoskeletal health, and sexual wellness. Originating from healthy, young donors and free of genetic material, exosomes offer a safe and powerful option for enhancing tissue regeneration and boosting overall health and function. For many of these treatments, however, patients may need to travel outside the United States.

Hair and Facial Cosmetic Rejuvenation: Localized, Targeted Exosome Treatments

When it comes to aesthetics, exosomes are proving to be a breakthrough in nonsurgical facial rejuvenation and for hair regrowth. In many ways, exosomes go beyond traditional methods of cosmetic treatments such as fillers or Botox, as they work on a cellular level to promote collagen production, reduce inflammation, and stimulate skin repair. The exosomes used in these cosmetic treatments are often derived from umbilical cord stem cells, rich in growth factors and proteins that support skin health. For better results, I design a customized program composed of a series of treatments over few weeks that integrates these exosome treatments with other modalities, such as PRP, dermal fillers, and laser treatments.

In procedures like *microneedling with exosomes*, the tiny punctures created in the skin allow the exosomes to penetrate deeply and deliver their growth factors more effectively, leading to faster healing, increased collagen production, and noticeable improvements in skin texture. For patients seeking natural, long-lasting rejuvenation without downtime, exosome therapy offers a promising alternative to traditional cosmetic procedures.

Exosome therapy can restore hair growth, skin elasticity, reduce the appearance of fine lines and wrinkles, and improve skin tone, offering a more youthful and natural appearance. Patients love the idea that these treatments aren't just masking signs of aging— they're actually rejuvenating their skin from the inside out. Based on the overwhelmingly positive outcomes the patients report, I believe that local exosome therapy represents a major breakthrough in the field of hair restoration, facial rejuvenation, and anti-aging medicine.

Musculoskeletal Health: Localized, Targeted Exosome Treatments

In the field of musculoskeletal health, exosomes are offering new hope for patients with chronic pain, joint degeneration, and sports injuries, much like the autologous stem cell injections we discussed earlier. One of the primary advantages of exosomes is their strong anti-inflammatory properties, which make them highly effective for conditions like osteoarthritis, tendinitis, and muscle injuries. For many patients, these conditions involve persistent inflammation and tissue degeneration, but exosome therapy can target the problem at the cellular level, reducing inflammation, promoting tissue repair, and stimulating the body's natural healing processes.

In many clinics across Europe and South America, exosomes are combined with other regenerative therapies, such as **PRP** or stem cells, to enhance healing and recovery for patients with joint injuries or degeneration. This approach is particularly beneficial for patients experiencing significant pain and limited mobility but who wish to avoid surgery. Whether it's an injured athlete recovering from a torn ligament or an older patient managing arthritis, exosomes offer a pathway to faster recovery and improved function.

In these procedures, exosomes can be injected directly into the affected joint, ligament, or tendon, where they work to repair damaged tissues and reduce chronic inflammation. Patients often report not only pain relief but also gains in mobility and strength, leading to a markedly improved quality of life.

Sexual Health—Localized, Targeted Exosome Treatments

One of the rapidly expanding uses of exosome therapy is in sexual health, particularly for treating erectile dysfunction (ED) in men. As with other conditions, exosomes enhance cellular communication and stimulate tissue repair in the local area. For ED, exosomes are injected directly into the cavernous tissue, where they promote angiogenesis (the formation of new blood vessels) and tissue regeneration, resulting in improved local blood flow.

For men struggling with ED due to aging, diabetes, or other health issues, exosome therapy provides a safe, regenerative alternative to more invasive treatments like implant surgery. Many patients who haven't responded to medications or other treatments have experienced significant improvements following exosome therapy. For these men, reclaiming their sexual health and confidence has been transformative.

Beyond ED, exosome therapy is also being explored in female sexual health to improve local tissue health, enhance sensitivity, and support regeneration. The regenerative effects of exosomes hold promise for improving sexual wellness in both men and women, addressing the underlying causes of dysfunction by repairing and rejuvenating tissues.

As we close this chapter, it's hard not to feel awe at the transformative potential of stem cells and exosomes for enhancing health and longevity. These therapies give us a glimpse into what it truly means to regenerate from within—not just to manage diseases but to reverse some of the damage that comes with aging. Their ability to restore vitality, rebuild tissues, and modulate the immune system opens doors that traditional medicine could never unlock.

But this journey does not stop here. As remarkable as these regenerative therapies are, in the next chapter, we'll explore a new frontier: psychedelics. Long misunderstood, these therapies are gaining attention for their ability to heal the mind, with implications that go far beyond treating depression or anxiety. These therapies may hold the key to enhancing longevity, building emotional resilience, supporting neuroplasticity, and unlocking new dimensions of health and well-being. Let's continue our journey into the next chapter, where the exploration of the mind meets the science of brain health.

CHAPTER 10

Psychedelics in Rejuvenation and Healing

> The world we live in is a mere reflection of the underlying reality, as seen through the filters of our senses.
> —The Doors of Perception, Aldous Huxley, British writer and philosopher (1894–1963)

> If the doors of perception were cleansed, everything would appear to man as it is, Infinite.
> —The Marriage of Heaven and Hell, William Blake, British poet and painter (1757–1827)

In the summer of 2023, as the sun dipped below the horizon, painting the sky in the shades of lavender and gold, the enchanting city of Bend, Oregon, came alive with possibilities. Nestled at the eastern foothills of the majestic Cascade Mountains, the rich scent of pine and the sweet fragrance of wildflowers permeated the air. The gentle rush of the Deschutes River provided a soothing soundtrack, its waters glistening as they meandered through the lush landscape.

In a secluded clearing surrounded by towering ponderosa pines, a group of adventurers gathered, their hearts beating with anticipation. Among them was a wise guide, a man deeply connected to the land and its ancient traditions. With a gentle smile, he revealed a small pouch of dried psilocybin mushrooms, a sacred medicine known for its mind-expanding properties. As he began to chant softly, his voice resonating with the rhythm of the natural world, the group felt a sense of calm wash over them.

The atmosphere shifted dramatically within thirty minutes of that first bite of the earthy mushroom. The vibrant greens of the forest seemed to pulse with a living energy, and the river, once a mere trickle, transformed into a shimmering ribbon of light. Others felt a oneness with the earth, as if the very ground beneath them was vibrating with the heartbeat of life itself. As the moon rose higher, its silvery glow illuminated the surroundings, revealing a tapestry of stars that felt intimately close, each twinkling light igniting a sense of wonder and connection.

Within minutes of the first taste of the earth-grown sacrament, reality began its magnificent transformation. For Sarah, the shift began in her fingertips: electric tingles of energy that spread through her body like liquid light. The forest floor beneath her began to pulse with bioluminescent patterns, each pine needle glowing with its own inner fire. Her consciousness expanded like ripples on still water, each wave carrying her farther from the shores of ordinary perception.

Michael felt it first in his chest: a flowering warmth that dissolved years of grief and guardedness. The trees around him began to dance with visible energy, their auras merging into rivers of green and gold light. Each breath drew in not just air but also liquid wisdom, filling every cell with the forest's ancient knowing. Tears flowed freely as his heart cracked open to a love larger than his personal story.

A young woman named Lily looked up at the sky, her breath catching in her throat as she perceived constellations dancing before her eyes. She felt an overwhelming connection to the ancient peoples who roamed these lands, their spirits lingering in the whispering breeze. The trees around her swayed gently, as if acknowledging her presence, and the earth beneath her feet throbbed with the rhythm of the cosmic heartbeat—a reminder of the intricate web of life.

Nearby, Jake, a middle-aged man burdened by the weight of daily responsibilities, stared into the crackling campfire. The flames twisted and turned, weaving stories of transformation. As the psilocybin took hold, he felt the tension in his shoulders dissipate, replaced by a profound sense of peace. Memories of lost opportunities and unfulfilled dreams floated to the surface, but instead of sorrow, he experienced a deep understanding—a realization that every moment had led him to this sacred gathering.

As the night deepened, the group settled into a shared silence, each person lost in his or her own heavenly voyage. The sounds of the forest—the rustle of leaves, the distant hoot of an owl, the soft burble of the river—became a symphony of connection. Each sound resonated with meaning, a reminder that they were part of something much larger than themselves.

With every heartbeat, they felt the essence of the trees and the earth come alive, each ancient root and leaf whispering secrets of resilience and unity. The very air around them seemed to vibrate with energy, and they were no longer just individuals but integral threads woven into the fabric of nature. They experienced a profound sense of oneness, as if the forest were breathing with them, and they were merging with the spirit of the land.

The guide, with his calm demeanor, observed the transformative experiences unfolding around the fire. He knew that these moments would weave through their lives, shaping their understanding of existence. These explorers, who sought adventure in the picturesque landscapes of Bend, were now partaking in something far greater: a collective awakening rooted in the power of psilocybin.

When dawn finally began to paint the eastern sky, it wasn't just light returning—it was as if the universe itself were being born anew. Each dewdrop contained galaxies, each bird's morning song carried codes of creation, and the rising sun bathed them all in waves of love so tangible it brought on fresh tears of gratitude.

The group would leave this place changed forever. They might not fully grasp the depths of their experience, but the feeling of unity with nature would resonate within them. This journey had evolved beyond mere exploration: it had become a sacred connection to the land, a testament to the healing power of the natural world, and it had become a journey into the depths of their own souls, forever intertwined with the beauty of Bend, Oregon. From then on, they would find themselves in the midst of something far greater: a moment of spiritual awakening, rooted in the sacred traditions of the land and the powerful medicine of the psilocybin mushrooms.

This wasn't just a night in Bend's embrace—it was a remembrance of humanity's place in the cosmic dance, a glimpse of the living poetry that underlies all reality, a journey into the very heart of existence itself. They carried within them now the unshakable knowledge that they were not separate observers of the universe, but were part of the universe itself, experiencing the miracle of its own unfolding through human eyes, hearts, and consciousness.

The Transcendent Mind

The experience of that group of adventurers in Bend is far from unique. The profound impact of psychedelic experiences on human consciousness continues to emerge as one of medicine's most fascinating frontiers. Through careful clinical observation and expanding scientific research, we're witnessing how these compounds can fundamentally alter our understanding of consciousness and perception. The experiences reported across diverse populations—from therapeutic settings to controlled research environments—reveal remarkably consistent patterns that challenge our conventional understanding of reality and consciousness.

> What intrigues me most is how individuals from vastly diverse backgrounds—using various psychedelic compounds, under varying circumstances, and across different eras—consistently describe similar transcendent experiences that transcend our ordinary sensory boundaries.

These experiences typically manifest as profound shifts in consciousness—from heightened sensory awareness to deep spiritual insights—suggesting access to aspects of reality typically filtered out by our everyday consciousness. Clinical studies demonstrate increasingly how these experiences can lead to lasting positive changes in personality, perspective, and emotional well-being.

The consistent reports of universal love, profound peace, and cosmic unity deserve serious scientific consideration. From Silicon Valley executives to military veterans, from cancer patients to mental health professionals, these experiences consistently transcend ordinary perceptual boundaries. What makes this particularly fascinating is how modern neuroscience is beginning to unravel the underlying mechanisms—showing how these substances can temporarily alter default-mode networks in the brain, potentially allowing access to broader realms of consciousness typically filtered out in our normal state.

These experiences suggest that our standard five-sense reality may represent just a narrow spectrum of available consciousness—much like a radio tuned to a single frequency among many. The therapeutic potential of these carefully guided experiences continues to demonstrate promising results in addressing conditions ranging from treatment-resistant depression to end-of-life anxiety, suggesting profound implications for mental health and human potential.

The integration of these experiences into therapeutic frameworks represents a significant advancement in mental health treatment. Research centers at prestigious institutions are documenting remarkable success rates in treating previously intractable conditions. The combination of psychedelic experiences with proper therapeutic support often catalyzes profound healing and personal transformation. What's particularly noteworthy is the durability of these changes, with many participants reporting sustained positive outcomes months and even years after their experiences.

Understanding the mechanism of action helps explain these sustained benefits. These therapeutic compounds appear to enhance *neuroplasticity* (the brain's capacity to adapt and change), potentially allowing the brain to break free from rigid thought patterns and establish healthier neural pathways. This *biological reset*, combined with the profound psychological insights gained during the experience, creates an optimal condition for lasting therapeutic change.

Psychedelics Use Since the Ancient Times

For millennia, psychedelics have been deeply woven into the cosmic, spiritual, and healing practices of cultures around the world. Let me share with you something profound from my experience as a medical practitioner as well as from this deep study of both ancient healing traditions and modern neuroscience. The transformative experiences we're seeing in places like Bend aren't isolated phenomena—they're part of humanity's oldest healing traditions, now validated by cutting-edge research.

Also, when I read about experiences of people in medical journals as well as in public writings, or when they share their stories with me, their experiences echo across time and culture. Whether it's a tech executive who found clarity in Bend's pine forests, a trauma survivor who experienced deep healing in a Peruvian ayahuasca ceremony, or an artist who rediscovered her creativity through guided psilocybin work in the Netherlands, I see consistent patterns of healing and awakening that align perfectly with both ancient wisdom and modern neuroscience.

The ancient use of psychedelic substances has deep roots in human history, with archaeological evidence suggesting their use for spiritual and healing purposes dating back thousands of years. Archaeological evidence shows us that sacred mushrooms were used in healing ceremonies as far back as 10,000 BC. In the prehistoric Sahara, rock art from around 7000 BC depicts mushrooms with psychedelic properties. In ancient Greece, the revered Eleusinian Mysteries—an annual religious festival lasting almost two millennia—may have centered on the consumption of a psychoactive drink called *kykeon*, believed to provide initiates with mystical experiences that transformed their understanding of life and death.

Similarly, indigenous cultures in Central and South America have long integrated psilocybin mushrooms and other psychedelic compounds into their spiritual and ritualistic practices. In ancient Mesoamerica, tribes like the Aztecs and the Maya used psilocybin mushrooms and peyote, rich in hallucinogen mescaline, to connect with the divine and experience transformative visions of the spiritual world. The Aztecs called psilocybin mushrooms *teonanácatl*—literally "flesh of the gods." Similarly, in the rainforests of South America, ayahuasca—a potent brew containing the psychedelic dimethyltryptamine (DMT)—has been central to shamanic traditions for centuries, offering physical healing and pathways to higher consciousness.

These early uses of psychedelics showcase the long-standing human quest to transcend ordinary reality and tap into deeper truths about existence. What fascinates me, as someone bridging traditional healing with modern medicine, is how these ancestral practices are now being validated by our most sophisticated research tools.

Now fast-forward to the mid-twentieth century, when psychedelics resurfaced in the Western world, spurred largely by the discovery of lysergic acid diethylamide (LSD) by Swiss chemist Albert Hofmann in 1938. By the 1960s, substances such LSD and psilocybin had become symbols of spiritual awakening and social revolution during the counterculture movement. However, widespread concerns over misuse and societal upheaval led to their criminalization by the late 1960s, effectively halting research and pushing these powerful substances into the shadows.

Yet psychedelics have since undergone a renaissance, returning not as mere hallucinogens but rather as powerful tools for mental health treatment and healing. Prestigious institutions such as Johns Hopkins University, Yale University, New York University, and Stanford University have spearheaded groundbreaking research highlighting the potential of psychedelics in treating conditions such as depression, PTSD, anxiety, incurable diseases, and addiction. Administered in controlled settings, these substances have been shown to foster profound psychological healing, enhance neuroplasticity, and promote long-term emotional well-being. The FDA has even granted breakthrough therapy status to psilocybin for treating major depression, highlighting its potential to revolutionize mental healthcare.

> Is it all just a funky dance of brain chemicals or some kind of true awakening to the transcendental realm beyond our five senses?

One of the most iconic moments in the history of psychedelics occurred in 1957, when R. Gordon Wasson, a curious New York banker, traveled to the mountains of southern Mexico to partake in an ancient psilocybin mushroom ceremony led by the revered native Mazatec shaman healer Maria Sabina Magdalena García from Huautla de Jiménez, Oaxaca, Mexico. For centuries, Maria and her people had used these "holy children" to connect with the divine and heal the mind and body. A day later, Valentina, a pediatrician and the wife of Wasson, decided to join him, along with their eighteen-year-old daughter, Masha.

Together, they partook in the enchanted mushrooms, each falling into a tapestry of vivid hallucinations. It was Valentina who had sowed the seeds of fascination for the so-called magic mushrooms in her husband's heart.

Wasson's transformative experience, which he recounted in a lengthy article in *Life* magazine titled " Seeking the Magic Mushroom", ignited widespread interest in psychedelics across the West. This pivotal moment sparked not just curiosity but also the realization that psychedelics could do more than open minds—*they might have the power to heal emotional wounds, treat mental disorders, and perhaps even reverse aspects of aging.*

People started to flock to Huautla de Jiménez to experience the psychedelic wonders. Timothy Leary, an American psychologist and author recognized for his passionate endorsement of psychedelic drugs, was among the notable figures who sought out Maria's healing rituals. Richard Alpert, another American psychologist, later widely known as Ram Dass, was equally intrigued by Wasson's accounts and visited to experience Sabina's ceremonies firsthand.

While the path of psychedelics has been complex—rising to prominence, falling under prohibition, and now reemerging with scientific credibility—their potential to heal and transform remains as powerful as ever. Today these ancient tools are finally being embraced by modern medicine, bringing the story of psychedelics full circle—from ancient spiritual rites to cutting-edge medical breakthroughs.

Through the Doorways of Consciousness: The Convergence of Three Transcendental States

Let me now take you on another journey that I find very intriguing and enchanting: *exploring the depths of our own self by examining three apparently distinct and unrelated paths.* I have long found it awe-inspiring that in the depths of human experience, these three paths wind their way toward the same ineffable summit. Like rivers flow-ing from distant springs, they converge in a sea of universal truth that has left seekers throughout the ages breathless with wonder.

First, there are those who have journeyed through the molecule-shaped doorways of psychedelics, their consciousness suddenly thrust into realms beyond ordinary perception. They speak of dissolving boundaries, of merging with an infinite cosmic dance, of encountering a love so vast it makes our earthly definitions seem like shadows cast by candlelight. Time loses its arrow; space sheds its rigid walls. They return with tears streaming down their faces, insisting that all is one, that death is but a mask worn by transformation, that consciousness itself is the fundamental fabric of reality.

Then there are those who have stood at the threshold between life and death, their bodies failing while their awareness expands beyond all known horizons. They float above operating tables or accident scenes, watching with strange serenity as medical teams fight for their lives. They speak of moving through tunnels of light, of encountering beings of pure radiance, of experiencing a review of their entire lives in a timeless instant. They too return transformed, their fear of death dissolved, their priorities fundamentally reordered by a glimpse of what waits beyond the veil.

And then, reaching across millennia, we hear the voices of the ancient rishis, all those Buddhas eons ago, those forest- and mountain-dwelling sages of India who turned their awareness inward with the precision of master surgeons. Deep in their meditation, they discovered the same vast, unending territories of consciousness, mapped the same ineffable geographies of spirit. In the Upanishads, a series of Hindu sacred treatises written in Sanskrit (circa 800–200 BC), they left us breadcrumbs leading to that same summit: "*Tat tvam asi*"—"That thou art." The individual self dissolves into the universal Self, the drop returning to the ocean while somehow retaining its "dropness."

I have pondered long and deeply—how is it that these three distinct paths, separated by substance, circumstance, cultures, and centuries, lead their travelers to such strikingly similar revelations? What are we to make of these overlapping maps drawn by such different cartographers? Are we seeing the same territory through different windows? Or different territories that just happen to inspire the same descriptions? As one of my friends says: *Is it all just a funky dance of brain chemicals or true awakening?*

Perhaps these experiences are like light passing through various prisms, each refracting the same fundamental truth through the particular angles of its approach. The psychedelic journeyer, the near-death survivor, and the meditation master may be like blind men touching different parts of the same cosmic elephant—each describing his local experience of a reality too vast for any single perspective to encompass and be able to describe.

To me, it seems that these convergent experiences are like paths drawn by different explorers who have climbed different faces of the same mountain peak—Chomolungma, as local Tibetans call it, or Mount Everest, as it is commonly known. Though their tracks varied, they all described the same breathtaking view from the summit—a view that hints at the possibility that consciousness itself might be far vaster and more mysterious than our ordinary experience suggests.

> How is it that these three separate paths, separated by substance, circumstance, cultures, and centuries, lead their travelers to such strikingly similar revelations? Is it simply some hidden area of the brain becoming active? Or are they peeking through some cosmic window and getting a glimpse of a broader reality beyond what we know with our five senses?

I had been thinking that what they might share is an irresistible conviction that our everyday consciousness is but the surface of an unfathomably deep ocean of infinite Intelligence all around us. They return with a common refrain: that love is the fundamental force of the universe, that death is not the end, that separation is an illusion, and that the nature of reality is far more mysterious and meaningful than our ordinary minds can grasp.

I strongly believe these commonalities whisper of something profound about the architecture of universes and consciousness itself. Like explorers returning from the same undiscovered country by different routes, their overlapping testimonies suggest that, when human awareness pushes beyond its ordinary boundaries, it encounters consistent features of a larger reality—one that always existed right here next to us and has been waiting patiently for us to notice it all along.

In their convergence, I find that these experiences challenge our assumptions about the nature of the mind, reality, and human potential. They hint at the possibility that consciousness itself may be more fundamental than we imagine—*not an emergent property of matter, but perhaps the very ground of being from which matter itself emerges.* They suggest that the mystics' poetic metaphors of unity might be more literally true than we supposed. Maybe we are those eternal beings whose "death" is only the beginning of that next adventure.

As we stand here in the twenty-first century, armed with both ancient wisdom and modern neuroscience, these questions beckon us toward deeper exploration. The striking similarities between these different paths of transcendence might be more than mere coincidence—they might be signposts pointing toward aspects of consciousness and reality that we are only beginning to understand. They challenge us to hold space for mystery and doubt, while maintaining our discerning intelligence and logic. Most of all, they suggest that the great philosophers' injunction to "know thyself" may lead us not just inward but also outward to the very edges of what we thought possible—and beyond.

Journeys of the Rich and Famous

When Prince Harry's memoir *Spare* hit bookstore shelves in 2023, revealing his profound healing experiences with psychedelics to cope with grief and loss, it marked more than just another celebrity headline. It represented a full-circle moment in humanity's relationship with these sacred medicines—a journey stretching from ancient ceremonial spaces to today's headlines and cutting-edge research labs.

Some other influential figures of our time are also helping to reintroduce these ancient practices to modern consciousness. Consider boxer Mike Tyson's remarkable transformation. The former heavyweight champion, once known for his intensity in the ring, describes how psilocybin and 5-MeO-DMT (a variant of dimethyltryptamine) helped him find profound peace. "My ego died," he's shared, a phrase that would resonate with both ancient shamans and modern neuroscientists studying the default-mode network. Today Iron Mike channels his passion into exploring psychedelic treatments for traumatic brain injury.

The influence of the late Steve Jobs on our modern world is undeniable, but less known is the Apple cofounder's statement that taking LSD was "one of the most important things in my life." This mirrors what Johns Hopkins and Imperial College London researchers are now discovering: that these compounds can enhance creativity and problem-solving by increasing neural plasticity and connectivity across typically isolated brain regions.

In the sports world, National Football League quarterback Aaron Rodgers's story particularly illuminates the potential for personal and professional transformation. According to Rodgers, his experiences with ayahuasca in Peru led to not just back-to-back MVP seasons but, more importantly, enhanced his leadership skills and deeper connections with teammates. This echoes what ancient wisdom traditions have long taught—that healing the individual flows outward to heal the community.

The entertainment world offers equally compelling accounts. Comedian Chelsea Handler's work with ayahuasca to process family trauma, actress Kristen Bell's groundbreaking experience with psilocybin for depression, and actor Will Smith's profound ayahuasca journeys—all point to what research is validating: these medicines can catalyze deep psychological healing when used thoughtfully in proper settings.

What fascinates me as a devoted student of both ancient healing traditions and modern medicine is how consistently these experiences, whether in Bend's forests or Silicon Valley retreats, mirror what traditional healers have long known. The same elements valued by indigenous healers—preparation, intention, guided support, and integration—are now being validated by clinical research as crucial for therapeutic outcomes.

Even more compelling is how these public figures' experiences align with what is shown by a meta-analysis study in 2020: when these elements are present, positive changes in well-being can persist for years. Whether it's author-investor Tim Ferriss funding groundbreaking research at Johns Hopkins, or podcaster Joe Rogan hosting discussions that normalize these conversations for millions, these influential voices are helping bridge ancient wisdom and modern understanding.

What's emerging is a powerful convergence—ancient ceremonial knowledge, modern scientific validation, and prominent voices sharing authentic experiences of transformation. Actor Morgan Freeman advocates thoughtfully for psilocybin research. Elon Musk has spoken openly about psychedelics' potential for healing trauma and expanding consciousness. Even more fascinating are the stories of Silicon Valley innovators who've incorporated microdosing practices into their creative processes, though always emphasizing the importance of intention and proper guidance.

Each story adds another thread to this tapestry of understanding, helping to destigmatize these medicines and supporting what researchers are calling the *psychedelic renaissance*. We're witnessing a unique moment in history where indigenous wisdom, modern science, and popular culture are converging to reshape our understanding of healing and consciousness.

What these experiences reveal consistently—whether from ancient ceremonies, modern research labs, or celebrity accounts—is psychedelics' remarkable capacity to catalyze what we in integrative and functional medicine call *whole-system healing*. The improvements span physical, emotional, spiritual, and relational dimensions, suggesting that these medicines work at the fundamental level of human consciousness, just as traditional healers have long maintained.

This convergence of ancient wisdom, modern science, and influential voices isn't just changing how we view these medicines—it's opening new possibilities for healing in our modern world. As these stories continue to emerge, they build bridges between traditional knowledge and contemporary understanding, offering hope for new approaches to mental health, creativity, and human potential.

Current Research with Psychedelic Compounds

Because of my curiosity and deep interest in this field, I have been following the evolving research in psychedelics. There are several natural and synthetic psychedelic compounds currently being researched for their potential therapeutic benefits in mental health, neuroplasticity (*rewiring of neural pathways in brain*), and neurogenesis (*generation and development of new functional neurons in the adult brain*). While none have full FDA approval yet for general use, many are in various phases of clinical trials for treating mental health disorders, including depression, anxiety, PTSD, and addiction.

- **Psilocybin (Natural):** Derived from so-called magic mushrooms, psilocybin is being studied extensively for its role in treating major depressive disorder, anxiety, PTSD, and addiction. Several clinical trials are ongoing, and psilocybin is expected to receive FDA approval in the near future for therapeutic use. It works by affecting serotonin receptors in the brain, promoting neuroplasticity and emotional healing.

- **DMT (Synthetic and Natural)**: N,N-Dimethyltryptamine is closely related to psilocybin, but it is a faster-acting psychedelic with effects on mental health outcomes. Commonly used as ayahuasca in Peru, it can produce an intense, acute experience that includes vivid visual imagery. It is present in a variety of plants and animals around the globe. 5-Methoxy-N,N-Dimethyltryptamine (5-MeO-DM), derived from the secretion of toads or synthesized, is currently being studied for its potential in treating depression and anxiety. Its short-acting nature combined with its ability to induce intense mystical experiences makes it a unique candidate in mental health treatments.
- **MDMA (Synthetic)**: Commonly known as Ecstasy or Molly, 3,4-methylenedioxymethamphetamine is in advanced clinical trials for the treatment of post-traumatic stress disorder. Unlike classic psychedelics, MDMA is classified as an *empathogen*, meaning that it enhances feelings of emotional connection and empathy. Its FDA approval is expected within the next few years, as it has shown significant promise in reducing PTSD symptoms in conjunction with psychotherapy.
- **Lysergic Acid Diethylamide (LSD) (Synthetic)**: LSD, another classic psychedelic, has a long history of use but is currently being revisited for its potential to treat anxiety, depression, and cluster headaches. Research on LSD's effects on neurogenesis and brain plasticity shows promise in improving cognitive flexibility and emotional resilience.
- **Ketamine (Synthetic)**: Ketamine, particularly its derivative esketamine (brand name, Spravato), has already

received FDA approval for treatment-resistant depression. It is also being researched for its potential in treating PTSD, suicidal ideation, and other mental health conditions. Ketamine works by affecting glutamate pathways and promoting rapid changes in neuroplasticity to bring about fast-acting antidepressant effects.

Legal Status and Current State of Approval of Psychedelics

There is huge amount of scientific data already available since the 1960s. Also, there is a tremendous amount of clinical research currently underway in academic institutions around the world and by many start-up companies. Yet, for reasons not quite clear to me, most psychedelics, including psilocybin and MDMA, are still not considered safe and are classified as Schedule I substances by the US Drug Enforcement Administration (DEA), meaning they are deemed to have no accepted medical use under US law and a high potential for abuse. However, ongoing clinical trials show promise in paving the way for FDA approval, particularly for psilocybin and MDMA in treating PTSD and depression.

After meticulously reviewing years of research, I do believe that, when prescribed judiciously, these psychedelic compounds offer a new dawn of hope for treating mental health disorders. From PTSD and depression to anxiety, brain injuries, end-of-life care, and numerous neurodegenerative illnesses, these substances enhance neuroplasticity, neurogenesis, and elevate overall emotional and psychological well-being.

I would like to add that the story of psychedelics being classified as Schedule I substances is deeply intertwined with the political and cultural landscape of 1960s America. Prior to their classification in 1970, psychedelics, particularly LSD, were the subject of extensive scientific research throughout the 1950s and 1960s, with promising therapeutic applications being studied in medical settings.

The Controlled Substances Act of 1970, signed into law under President Richard Nixon, drastically changed the landscape by classifying psychedelics as Schedule I substances. This classification was ostensibly based on three criteria: a high potential for abuse, no currently accepted medical use, and a lack of accepted safety under medical supervision.

However, the historical context reveals a more complex picture. The classification coincided with the height of the counterculture movement and young people's increasingly vehement protests against the protracted Vietnam War. Psychedelics had become symbolic of cultural rebellion. The decision was influenced little by medical considerations and more so by political reactions to the social upheaval of the time, coupled with media sensationalism about recreational use.

The Schedule I classification had far-reaching consequences, effectively halting most legitimate research into these compounds for decades. This decision notably contradicted existing research that had demonstrated therapeutic potential and relatively low abuse potential compared with other substances. Many researchers today agree that the classification was more influenced by political and social factors than by scientific evidence. The decision went against the recommendations of numerous medical professionals of the time, creating a decades-long pause in what had been a promising field of medical research.

However, many ongoing clinical trials, some of which are in late stages, are paving the way for FDA approval, particularly for psilocybin and MDMA in the treatment of PTSD and depression. The states of Oregon and Colorado now permit limited availability of psilocybin under strict regulatory guidelines. We need to keep an eye on this rapidly evolving landscape as more clinical trial data emerge.

Diseases Impacted by Psychedelics

What excites me is the fact that psychedelics are so remarkable in their ability to go beyond mere symptom management. Unlike conventional medications that only numb or suppress symptoms, psychedelics offer a deeply transformative experience—one that allows individuals to confront trauma, process grief, and gain insights that can reshape their emotional and psychological outlook. Psilocybin and ketamine have shown incredible promise in treating *end-of-life care, PTSD, brain injuries, anxiety, treatment-resistant depression, prolonged grief, and addiction.* Patients often describe the experience as a rebirth—a moment of awakening where they reconnect with life and break free from the heavy burdens that have weighed them down for years, even decades.

But perhaps the most exciting part of this new psychedelic frontier isn't just in mental health—it's in the realm of longevity and anti-aging. Beyond their ability to heal the mind, psychedelics are now being explored for their role in neuroplasticity, the brain's ability to rewire and regenerate. Studies are showing that psychedelics may stimulate neurogenesis, promoting the growth of new neurons and helping to repair the brain's pathways. This has profound implications for age-related cognitive decline and neurodegenerative diseases such as Alzheimer's and Parkinson's. Could psychedelics hold the key to preserving mental sharpness well into old age? The early research suggests they might.

Moreover, psychedelics may play a crucial role in reducing chronic inflammation, which, as you know, is one of the primary drivers of aging. Chronic inflammation not only accelerates the aging process but also contributes to a host of diseases, from heart disease to diabetes. By reducing inflammation and promoting cellular regeneration, psychedelics could offer a pathway to disease reversal and healing. Imagine a treatment that helps restore your mind while also rejuvenating your body, helping you not only live longer but live better.

These discoveries are not just speculative—they are being backed by rigorous science. Johns Hopkins recently published groundbreaking studies showing that psilocybin can produce lasting changes in mood and cognition, while New York University is exploring how these substances can help cancer patients confront their fear of death with peace and clarity. Stanford University's research delves into how ketamine can rapidly treat depression by rewiring the brain in ways that conventional treatments never could. Psychedelics are offering hope where conventional medicine has often fallen short.

Psychedelics are more than just mind-altering substances; they are a gateway to a new understanding of mental health, longevity, and human potential. From their sacred roots in indigenous cultures to their cutting-edge applications in modern medicine, psychedelics are emerging as powerful tools in the quest for a longer, healthier life. The future of medicine is not just about treating symptoms—it's about holistic healing, where the mind, body, and spirit are all aligned. And psychedelics may very well be the key to unlocking this next frontier in anti-aging and well-being.

More on Neuroplasticity and Neurogenesis

Our brains are magnificent engines of transformation, constantly growing new nerve cells (neurogenesis) and rewiring neural pathways (neuroplasticity). Let's dive into how these remarkable processes maintain our cognitive vitality. The hippocampus stands as a testament to the brain's regenerative power. Within this crucial memory center, new neurons spring to life throughout our existence. These fresh cells are vital architects of our memory formation, learning capacity, and emotional resilience. Think of it as our brain's perpetual renewal system, working tirelessly to maintain our cognitive edge.

Our neural networks are masters of adaptation, continuously morphing and evolving. Each experience we encounter, each skill we master, each challenge we face triggers a cascade of changes in our neural architecture. This incredible plasticity allows our brains to recover from injury, adapt to new circumstances, and evolve with every passing day. It's a testament to our inherent capacity for lifelong growth and adaptation.

The antiquated belief that our adult brains were static has crumbled in the face of modern neuroscience. We now know our brains remain wonderfully plastic and generative throughout life. Environmental enrichment, physical activity, and certain compounds—including psychedelics—can amplify these natural growth processes, tapping into our brain's innate regenerative capabilities. This revolutionary understanding illuminates exciting pathways for addressing cognitive decline, optimizing mental health, and potentially treating neurodegenerative conditions. Our brains harbor far more potential for growth and adaptation than previously imagined.

Neuroscientific research reveals intriguing patterns in brain activity during these psychedelic experiences. Advanced imaging studies demonstrate significant changes in neural connectivity, particularly in regions of the brain associated with self-awareness, emotional processing, and pattern recognition. The temporary disruption of the default-mode network—our brain's autopilot system—appears to allow novel connections and perspectives previously inaccessible to conscious awareness. This neuroplastic state can facilitate profound therapeutic breakthroughs, particularly in cases where traditional therapeutic approaches have reached their limits.

> Neuroscience research shows that psychedelics provide a sort of biological neural reset from improved neuroplasticity and neurogenesis, with tremendous potential for helping people suffering from various illnesses.

The implications are profound: from enhancing our learning potential to recovering from injury to maintaining cognitive vitality as we age. By understanding and harnessing these natural processes, we can better support our brain's remarkable capacity for renewal and adaptation.

Psychedelics and Their Role in Neurogenesis and Neuroplasticity

Psychedelics such as psilocybin, LSD, and ayahuasca are now being studied extensively for their potential to promote both neurogenesis and neuroplasticity. These compounds act on the serotonin 5-HT2A receptors in the brain, which play a key role in regulating mood, cognition, and neurogenesis. When these receptors are activated by psychedelics, they stimulate the production of *brain-derived neurotrophic factor (BDNF)*—a protein that supports the growth of new neurons and enhances synaptic connections.

BDNF is crucial for brain plasticity, particularly in areas of the brain responsible for memory and learning, like the hippocampus. Increased levels of BDNF have been associated with enhanced cognitive function, emotional resilience, and overall brain health. By facilitating the release of BDNF, psychedelics help the brain form new neural pathways and strengthen existing ones, effectively "rewiring" the brain. This can lead to significant improvements in cognitive flexibility, the ability to learn new things, adapt to changes, and overcome harmful patterns of thought—traits that are particularly beneficial in treating mental health conditions.

Research on Diseases Impacted by Improved Neurogenesis and Neuroplasticity

The ability of psychedelics to promote neurogenesis and neuroplasticity holds immense potential for treating a variety of diseases and disorders. Here are some of the key conditions that could benefit:

- **Depression and Anxiety:** One of the hallmarks of major depressive disorder (MDD) and chronic anxiety is impaired neurogenesis, particularly in the hippocampus. People with depression often show reduced hippocampal size, which is linked to cognitive deficits and emotional dysregulation. By promoting neurogenesis and enhancing neural plasticity, psychedelics offer a way to reverse this damage. The brain's ability to reorganize itself allows for healthier emotional processing and the breaking of negative thought patterns.
- **Post-Traumatic Stress Disorder:** PTSD is another condition characterized by dysfunctional neural circuitry, especially in areas of the brain involved in memory and emotional regulation, such as the *amygdala* and hippocampus. Psychedelics, particularly MDMA (although not traditionally categorized with classic psychedelics like psilocybin, it works similarly in promoting neuroplasticity), have shown promise in facilitating emotional healing by helping the brain form new connections and process traumatic memories in a less emotionally charged manner. By enhancing neuroplasticity, these substances help individuals reframe their trauma and reduce the intensity of negative emotional responses.
- **Alzheimer's Disease and Cognitive Decline:** Neurodegenerative diseases such as Alzheimer's are marked by the loss of neurons and synaptic connections, leading to memory loss, cognitive decline, and other neurological impairments. While psychedelics are still in the early stages of research for these conditions, their ability to enhance neurogenesis and neuroplasticity offers hope for repairing damaged neural circuits and slowing the progression of these diseases. By promoting the formation of new neurons and improving synaptic plasticity,

psychedelic therapies may help patients maintain cognitive function for longer periods.
- **Addiction:** Substance use disorders (a pattern of drug or alcohol use that persists despite negative consequences) are often driven by deeply ingrained neural pathways that reinforce cravings and compulsive behavior. Psychedelics such as ibogaine, psilocybin, and ayahuasca have shown potential in helping patients overcome addiction by promoting neuroplasticity and allowing the brain to rewire these maladaptive pathways. Studies suggest that these substances can disrupt the habitual thought patterns that drive addiction and offer a new perspective, making it easier for individuals to overcome substance dependence.
- **Traumatic Brain Injury (TBI):** These injuries can severely impair neurogenesis and neuroplasticity, leading to cognitive deficits, memory issues, and emotional dysregulation. Early research suggests that psychedelics might help promote neurogenesis and neural repair after a brain injury by stimulating BDNF and enhancing the brain's ability to form new connections. While more research is needed, the neuroplastic effects of psychedelics could eventually offer a novel approach to brain injury rehabilitation.

Overall, the ability of psychedelics to enhance neurogenesis and neuroplasticity represents a promising new frontier in neuroscience. By fostering the brain's ability to adapt and heal, psychedelics may hold the key to treating a wide range of mental health disorders and neurodegenerative conditions, ultimately improving both brain function and quality of life.

More on Psilocybin: "Magic Mushroom"

For the past several years, I have been closely following the rapidly evolving landscape around psilocybin, driven by deep personal conviction in its vast potential. My intensive study encompasses both the rigorous preclinical and clinical trials revealing its therapeutic power and the complex regulatory landscape shaping its future. This stems from my firm belief in psilocybin's capacity to revolutionize mental healthcare, treat diseases, and influence human longevity. The emerging research data continues to strengthen my commitment to following this field's rapid evolution.

Psilocybin, the active compound found in certain species of mushrooms, is experiencing a groundbreaking resurgence in the medical world. What was once dismissed as a counterculture drug is now being hailed as one of the most promising tools for mental health and emotional healing. Johns Hopkins University, NYU, and Imperial College London are leading the charge in psilocybin research, exploring its profound effects on conditions such as *depression, anxiety, and addiction, as well as its use in end-of-life care*. The results have been nothing short of transformative, paving the way for a new era of psychedelic-assisted therapies.

One of the most notable areas where psilocybin is making waves is in end-of-life care. Patients facing terminal illnesses often experience debilitating anxiety, fear, and depression as they come to terms with their mortality. Traditional treatments—like antidepressants—often fall short, leaving these individuals emotionally paralyzed. Enter psilocybin. Clinical trials at Johns Hopkins and NYU have shown that a single dose of psilocybin, administered in a controlled, therapeutic setting, can lead to profound and lasting reductions in anxiety and depression for patients confronting death. These patients often describe the experience as spiritually liberating, allowing them to reconnect with a deeper sense of meaning and acceptance in their final days. (In case you are interested in enrolling in any currently active trial worldwide, visit the US National Institutes of Health website ClinicalTrials.gov.)

But the power of psilocybin doesn't stop there. It's also showing incredible promise in treating *emotional disorders like depression and anxiety*, particularly in cases where traditional treatments have failed. Studies have shown that psilocybin can help reset the brain's default-mode network, which is often hyperactive in those with depression and anxiety. This reboot allows patients to break free from negative thought patterns, giving them the emotional clarity and mental space to heal. Unlike conventional antidepressants, which can take weeks to show effects and often require long-term use, psilocybin offers rapid, long-lasting benefits after just one or two therapeutic sessions.

Another area of exploration is the use of psilocybin in treating *addiction*. Studies at Johns Hopkins have found that psilocybin can significantly reduce cravings and help patients struggling with substance use disorders, particularly in smoking and alcohol addiction. By helping individuals access suppressed emotions and past traumas, psilocybin allows them to confront the root causes of their addiction and take meaningful steps toward recovery. The deep, introspective experiences often facilitated by psilocybin have been described as life-changing, with many participants reporting a newfound sense of purpose and control over their lives.

Psilocybin is also gaining attention for its potential role in treating *brain injuries and other brain disorders*. Early studies suggest that psilocybin may promote the brain's ability to rewire and heal itself. This is particularly promising for individuals recovering from traumatic brain injuries, stroke, and other neurological conditions. By stimulating the growth of new neurons and enhancing the brain's natural healing process, psilocybin could become a vital tool in neurorehabilitation.

In 2020 Oregon became the first US state to legalize the therapeutic use of psilocybin with Measure 109, which allows licensed facilitators to administer psilocybin to individuals in supervised settings for therapeutic purposes. This groundbreaking legislation marked a major shift in how psychedelics are viewed in terms of public health and mental health treatments.

Colorado followed closely behind and passed Proposition 122 in November 2022, decriminalizing the possession and use of certain psychedelics, including psilocybin. The state is now moving toward establishing a framework for psilocybin-assisted therapy, similar to Oregon's model. These legislative moves reflect the growing recognition of the therapeutic benefits of psilocybin, especially for treating mental health conditions such as depression, PTSD, anxiety, and addiction.

The growing acceptance of psychedelics at the state level could pave the way for broader use and further research into their potential benefits for mental health and longevity. It's a pivotal moment in the resurgence of psychedelic medicine.

As I see it, the current state of psilocybin research is incredibly promising, with dozens of clinical trials underway and mounting evidence of its potential to revolutionize how we approach mental health and healing. As the stigma around psychedelics continues to fade, and as more clinics integrate psilocybin-assisted therapy into their treatment offerings, we may be on the cusp of a new era—one where the mind's capacity for healing is unlocked in ways we never thought possible.

Ketamine: Its Evolving Role in Health and Longevity

Ketamine has an interesting history; it was originally developed in the 1960s as an anesthetic medicine for medical procedures. Known for its fast-acting and dissociative properties (a set of hallucinogenic effects that can include detachment from reality, hallucinations, and altered senses), it was widely used during the Vietnam War to treat injured soldiers on the battlefield. However, beyond its role as an anesthetic, researchers soon began noticing its potential for other uses. By the early 2000s, ketamine was being explored as a treatment for mental health conditions, particularly in patients for whom antidepressants and other traditional treatments had failed.

Today ketamine is making waves in the world of mental health and chronic pain management, with ketamine infusion clinics popping up across the country. One of its most remarkable effects is its ability to rapidly alleviate symptoms of depression and anxiety, often within hours or days—compared with traditional antidepressants, which can take weeks or even months. Ketamine works by blocking N-methyl-D-aspartate (NMDA) receptors in the brain. These receptors are glutamate-gated ion channels that play a key role in helping reset neural pathways. Ketamine thus enhances neuroplasticity, enabling the brain to rewire itself. This has been particularly effective in patients with treatment-resistant depression, where other medications have failed. Many patients report profound relief from long-standing symptoms after just a few ketamine sessions.

Clinical studies have associated the mental health improvements from ketamine with enhanced neuroplasticity and new synaptic connections in the brain. That is, ketamine therapy can help to get at the root cause of the psychological pain rather than just at the symptoms that arise as a result. Also, ketamine therapy, as an alternative treatment for depression and anxiety, doesn't carry the same side effect profile as more traditional antidepressants. For instance, the selective serotonin reuptake inhibitors (SSRIs) Prozac, Paxil, and Zoloft can bring about sexual side effects, weight gain, and emotional numbness. For people who've had difficulties with SSRIs, ketamine can provide an alternative option.

Ketamine is also used in the treatment of *chronic pain*, especially for patients trying to avoid addictive opioids. For patients suffering from neuropathic pain, fibromyalgia, or complex regional pain syndrome (CRPS), in which a chronic pain condition develops after an injury or surgery, typically affecting an arm or leg, ketamine infusions have shown significant promise in reducing pain levels. By interrupting pain signals in the nervous system, ketamine offers a potential solution for those whose pain has been unmanageable with other therapies. What makes ketamine particularly valuable in pain management protocols is its ability to relieve pain without the long-term side effects or addictive potential often seen with opioids, making it a safer alternative in the fight against chronic pain.

In addition to pain relief and mental health treatment, ketamine is gaining recognition in the field of *addiction recovery*. Clinical studies have found that ketamine can help reduce cravings and support long-term abstinence in patients struggling with alcohol or substance use disorders. Its ability to create a dissociative state allows patients to explore the underlying emotional issues that often fuel addiction, breaking cycles of dependency. Ketamine's unique neurochemical effects, combined with psychotherapy, can lead to lasting behavioral changes.

Ketamine is also showing potential for patients with *traumatic brain injuries*. Due to its neuroprotective properties and ability to promote neuroplasticity, the drug is being explored as a treatment to enhance brain recovery and improve cognitive function. In patients who have suffered TBIs, ketamine's effects on synaptic connections and the brain's healing processes may offer new hope for improved recovery outcomes.

For emotional disorders such as *anxiety, depression, and PTSD*, ketamine provides an alternative to traditional therapies that can sometimes take years to make an impact. In carefully monitored clinical settings, ketamine infusions can provide almost immediate relief from debilitating anxiety and PTSD symptoms, giving patients a window of clarity and peace that allows them to process trauma and move forward in their lives. Ketamine-assisted psychotherapy has been particularly effective in allowing individuals to confront and reframe deep emotional wounds that contribute to their condition.

Let me share my clinical experience with oral ketamine therapy, which has really transformed how I can help patients. In my practice, I've seen remarkable success using two distinct approaches. The first is *intermittent dosing protocols*, where we administer therapeutic doses three times a week. The second approach, which particularly excites me, is daily *microdosing or very-low-dose (VLD) therapy*. This gentler method works wonderfully for treating certain conditions such as *phobias, social anxiety, eating disorders, obsessive-compulsive disorder, and anxiety*. It has also shown intriguing potential for *anti-aging benefits*.

What's particularly intriguing about oral ketamine is how it's opened new possibilities for treatment. Unlike traditional infusions conducted in a clinical setting, the oral form offers much more flexibility. I've found this especially valuable for my patients who need ongoing support but prefer treatment in the comfort of their own homes. Of course, we have to maintain careful medical oversight throughout the course of treatment—*combining these treatments with counseling sessions to ensure both safety and optimal therapeutic benefit*. I've been consistently impressed by how this integrative approach helps unlock ketamine's full potential for mental health, chronic pain, and other challenging conditions. Through years of clinical experience, I've refined these protocols to be both safe and effective. It's incredibly rewarding to see how this more accessible form of ketamine therapy is helping people who previously had limited options.

Currently, ketamine is not yet widely recognized or researched specifically for its direct role in *anti-aging, youthfulness, or longevity*. Most of its therapeutic applications are focused on mental health, chronic pain, and addiction treatment. However, some indirect benefits related to its effects on mental well-being and neuroplasticity could potentially contribute to a better quality of life and healthier aging.

By improving mental health conditions like depression and anxiety, ketamine may help reduce chronic stress, which is a known factor in accelerated aging and poor overall health. Additionally, ketamine's ability to promote neuroplasticity could support cognitive health and resilience as we age. Enhanced neuroplasticity has been linked to maintaining cognitive function and potentially reducing the risk of neurodegenerative diseases that often come with aging, such as Alzheimer's and Parkinson's.

Although psychedelics, including ketamine, aren't yet recognized as direct anti-aging therapies by longevity experts, *I firmly believe they hold remarkable potential for promoting youthfulness, sharper thinking, and enhanced vitality in the right individuals.* Whether through episodic treatments or low-dose protocols, psychedelics' ability to boost mental health, reduce stress, and enhance cognitive flexibility supports holistic well-being, which is key to living a longer, healthier life. While more research is needed, the potential for psychedelics, including ketamine, in the anti-aging field is undeniably exciting.

While psychedelic therapy, including ketamine microdosing as used in VitalLife, is still in its early stages for direct benefits for longevity, by strengthening the mind-body connection, psychedelics like ketamine may offer a more holistic approach to aging, helping to maintain not only mental clarity but also emotional well-being and even physical rejuvenation.

I envision a future where these treatments are fully embraced, integrated into healthcare systems and accessible to those in need. A future where people suffering from mental health struggles can turn to these therapies safely and legally, with the guidance of medical professionals. It's a future filled with hope—a new path to healing that we are only beginning to explore, but one that holds immense potential for well-being and longevity.

As we move from the fascinating world of psychedelics, it's time to explore another powerful realm in the pursuit of longevity and youthfulness: hormones and peptides. These critical components of our body's natural chemistry play a fundamental role in everything from energy levels and sexual health to skin elasticity and muscle strength. By understanding how hormones and peptides can be optimized, we unlock new possibilities for slowing the aging process, enhancing performance, and restoring the youthful vibrancy that allows us to live healthier, longer lives.

CHAPTER 11

Optimizing Hormones and Peptides for Youthful Vitality

> To live is the rarest thing in the world. Most people just exist, that is all.
> —*Oscar Wilde, Irish writer (1854–1900)*

> The secret of staying young is to live honestly, eat slowly, and lie about your age.
> —*Lucille Ball, American comedian and actress (1911–1994)*

Renee was a forty-six-year-old TV personality whose vibrant, fast-paced life was turned upside down. For more than a year, Renee had been battling overwhelming fatigue, emotional sadness, and what she described as a constant brain fog. Her once restful nights were now restless, leaving her unable to sleep deeply. Desperate for answers, she sought help from her primary care physician, who ran some routine blood tests that were found to be normal, and, like so many, her physician diagnosed her with depression. She was prescribed Paxil, a common antidepressant. But instead of feeling better, Renee became more lethargic and disconnected from the life she once thrived in.

By the time she came to see me, Renee was tired in more ways than one. She had accepted that she might never feel like herself again. That this was just part of her getting older and something inevitable. But as I listened to her describe her struggles, it became clear that her symptoms were not just emotional. There was something deeper at play. After conducting a series of comprehensive biomarker tests—not just the standard blood work but a full hormonal and metabolic assessment—I saw that Renee's issues were rooted in a complex hormonal and peptide imbalance.

Based on her biomarker data and medical history, I crafted a personalized VitalLife treatment plan for her, starting with a customized hormone blend that included estrogen, progesterone, testosterone, pregnenolone, and thyroid hormone to restore her energy and mental clarity. Alongside this, I prescribed sermorelin, a peptide that encourages the body's natural production of growth hormone, to address her fatigue and support muscle recovery. To further boost her cellular energy, I added NAD+ therapy, a coenzyme that helps repair and energize cells. Coupled with these, Renee also received dietary modifications, support for her microbiome, and a range of supplements and herbs to restore her body's balance.

In less than six weeks, Renee was almost unrecognizable—her energy surged, she started sleeping soundly, and the brain fog lifted. She made the decision to stop taking Paxil on her own, feeling emotionally and physically better than she had in years. "It's like I've been given ten years of my life back," she told me, her smile wide and eyes bright, just like I had seen her when she is on her TV program. The transformation wasn't just physical; she felt empowered again, reconnected with her life and her passions.

I could fill volumes with stories like Renee's—transformations I've witnessed over the past twenty years that are nothing short of life-changing. It's not just about hormones or peptides; it's about giving people back the spark they need to feel alive again. And for me, as a healer and clinician, there's nothing more fulfilling than watching someone reclaim their life, watching their confidence return as they step into a new chapter of health and well-being. It's why I enjoy doing what I do, and it's what makes every moment of my work so rewarding.

Comprehensive Hormone Optimization, Not Hormone Replacement

Hormones are chemical messengers produced by various glands in the body, such as the thyroid, adrenal glands, and reproductive organs. These molecules regulate numerous bodily functions, from metabolism and mood to growth and reproduction. Essentially, they are the key drivers of many processes that keep us healthy and feeling energetic.

Peptides, on the other hand, are short chains of amino acids, smaller than proteins, that signal cells to perform specific tasks. In regenerative medicine and anti-aging therapies, peptides are often used to trigger processes such as tissue repair, collagen production, and even the stimulation of growth hormone—helping to restore youthfulness, energy, and vitality.

Imagine your hormones as a grand orchestra, performing nature's most sophisticated symphony. Just as Beethoven conducted his masterpieces with precise timing and perfect harmony, your endocrine system orchestrates an intricate dance of hormones that keeps you vibrant, energized, and youthful. In my years of practice, I've seen how even subtle disruptions in this delicate hormone symphony can ripple through your entire well-being.

Now let's talk about hormone and peptide optimization. *It is fundamentally different from conventional hormone replacement therapy offered at most hormone clinics and medspas.* Hormone optimization doesn't just aim to replace what's missing; it's about finding the right balance of various hormones to get your body functioning at its peak. In conventional hormone replacement therapy, patients are often given a standard dosage of hormones without much customization. This cookie-cutter approach lacks the personalization that hormone optimization provides. It assumes that everyone will benefit from the same treatment, but in reality, our bodies are much more complex.

Hormone optimization works by taking a comprehensive, scientific, and data-based approach to assess where your specific imbalances lie. The goal isn't just to get your hormone levels into a "normal range" but to adjust them, so they're optimized for your unique biology. This requires running a thorough panel of biomarker tests, which includes not only hormone levels but also markers for inflammation, metabolism, mitochondrial function, and more. These tests provide a clear picture of your body's internal environment, allowing for a personalized treatment plan.

These days I see an avalanche of testosterone and other hormone replacement programs offered by medspas and other hormone clinics, which can be bad if using a *cookie-cutter approach*, as most do. Based on my extensive experience in prescribing hormones and peptides, I can emphatically state that it's crucial to adopt a personalized and comprehensive holistic approach when offering hormones to individuals. Each hormone serves a unique function. Growth hormone supports cellular renewal and vitality. Testosterone and estrogen sustain strength, clarity, and zest. Oxytocin, often called the "love hormone," fosters emotional connection, intimacy, and an overall sense of well-being.

> Hormone optimization doesn't just "replace" what's missing—it helps restore your entire hormonal ecosystem. This approach is a personalized, comprehensive approach that uses a custom blend of synergistic hormones and peptides; metabolic, mitochondrial, and immune support; and lifestyle strategies for optimal results.

Adding peptides such as sermorelin, a growth hormone–releasing hormone (GHRH), that stimulate the body's own production of growth hormone, helps to improve sleep, energy levels, muscle tone, and overall recovery. Additionally, PT-141, a peptide used for enhancing sexual function, can further complement testosterone therapy by improving libido and erectile function, creating a synergistic effect that maximizes sexual vitality.

The difference here is that instead of a one-size-fits-all prescription, the VitalLife program emphasizes a *hormone and peptide optimization with tailored treatments to the individual's unique biological needs*. This kind of personalized approach leads to better outcomes because it targets the exact issues the person is experiencing—whether it's chronic fatigue, mood swings, muscle weakness, cognitive decline, or weight gain.

With VitalLife, I always take a comprehensive and personalized data-driven approach to hormone optimization, integrating not just testosterone or estrogen, but a range of hormones and peptides designed to address the full spectrum of aging and wellness. By carefully balancing these hormones, while also supporting key systems such as metabolism, gut health, and mitochondrial function, the program delivers tailored, evidence-based solutions for optimal health and longevity. By addressing these interconnected systems, you set the foundation for not just hormonal balance but also long-term vitality and health resilience. This is precision medicine at its finest, where each intervention is thoughtfully chosen to help you reclaim the energy, clarity, and vitality that time may have diminished.

Testosterone Optimization Therapy (TOT) in Men

Testosterone is a critical hormone that plays an essential role in a man's overall health, vitality, and well-being. As men age, testosterone levels naturally decline, leading to a range of physical, emotional, and cognitive changes that can significantly affect quality of life. Symptoms of testosterone deficiency, or low testosterone (*Low-T*), are often subtle at first but can worsen over time. Common symptoms include persistent fatigue, a decrease in muscle mass and strength, weight gain (particularly around the midsection), and a reduction in libido and sexual performance. Many men with low testosterone may also experience erectile dysfunction, difficulty maintaining an erection, or a diminished interest in sexual activity.

Beyond these physical changes, I have seen how low testosterone levels can also impact mental health, causing mood swings, irritability, feelings of depression, and a decline in cognitive function, often described as "brain fog." Additionally, testosterone deficiency can contribute to the loss of bone density, increasing the risk of fractures and osteoporosis, further complicating the aging process. These symptoms, though often mistaken as part of normal aging, can be effectively addressed through testosterone optimization, restoring vitality and reversing many of these undesired effects.

Prescribing Testosterone: The VitalLife Approach

When it comes to prescribing testosterone as part of VitalLife, instead of the one-size-fits-all approach of replacement prevalent these days (commonly called testosterone replacement therapy, or TRT), I prefer to use *testosterone optimization therapy* (TOT). As we discussed above, hormone optimization emphasizes a comprehensive hormone optimization approach instead of the knee-jerk reaction of prescribing testosterone injections alone without a comprehensive plan. It is essential to carefully *integrate hormones, estrogen blockers, and peptides with strategies for helping metabolism, the gut, and mitochondria.*

For TOT, there are several effective and customizable testosterone hormone options available. The four primary forms of injectable testosterone are testosterone enanthate, testosterone cypionate, testosterone propionate, and testosterone undecanoate. Each of these injectable forms has unique properties in terms of how long they remain active in the body, allowing for tailored dosing schedules depending on your medical needs and goals. In addition to these injections, testosterone can also be delivered through various alternative methods, such as *oral tablets, buccal tablets, transdermal gels, patches, solutions, and pellets implanted under the skin* for a long-lasting, steady release of the hormone. The method of administration is often selected based on individual preferences, convenience, lifestyle, and overall health considerations.

> For TOT, it is essential to carefully integrate hormones, estrogen blockers, and peptides with strategies for helping metabolism, the gut, and mitochondria.

The results of properly optimized testosterone are truly remarkable. I've witnessed profound transformations in countless men. The benefits seen are substantial and go beyond just symptom relief. Men who undergo TOT often report a dramatic increase in energy levels, improved muscle mass and strength, better fat distribution, and a sharper mental focus. Testosterone therapy can also enhance sexual function, restoring libido, improving erectile quality, and boosting confidence in intimate relationships. Additionally, many men experience an overall improvement in mood, reduced anxiety, and a sense of well-being and rejuvenation. By optimizing testosterone levels, men can experience not just a reversal of the symptoms of aging but a renewed sense of vitality and confidence, helping them live their lives with more vigor and purpose.

Side Effects and Precautions of Testosterone Hormone Therapy

Let me be clear: as with any other medical treatment, testosterone therapy is not for everyone. It is very important for you and your doctor to balance the benefits against possible risks for *you*. That's why a cookie-cutter approach and buying testosterone over the internet without proper physician supervision is very dangerous. Any testosterone therapy should be approached carefully and with a thorough understanding of the individual's overall health profile.

Some common side effects include increased red blood cell production (erythrocytosis), which can lead to a thickening of the blood and potentially increase the risk of blood clots, heart attacks, or strokes. It is essential to regularly monitor blood counts to mitigate these risks. Additionally, some men may experience acne, oily skin, or mood swings as hormone levels fluctuate, particularly when testosterone is not properly balanced with other hormones.

Another concern is that giving testosterone hormone to patients can lead to a decrease in testicular size (testicular atrophy) and reduced sperm production, which may impact fertility. This is because exogenous testosterone can suppress the body's natural production of testosterone and reduce the signaling hormones involved in sperm production. Men who are considering future family planning should discuss this thoroughly with their healthcare provider before starting any testosterone treatment. Sleep apnea is another condition that can worsen with testosterone therapy, and it's essential to screen for this condition beforehand, especially in men with a history of sleep issues or obesity.

Lastly, men with prostate cancer or those at high risk for developing it should typically avoid testosterone therapy, as it can stimulate the growth of prostate tissue. Men with severe heart conditions should also proceed with caution, as exogenous testosterone may exacerbate certain cardiovascular issues. Additionally, those with uncontrolled high blood pressure or a history of blood clots should be thoroughly evaluated to determine if the benefits of testosterone therapy outweigh the potential risks.

I believe that, while TOT can offer life-changing benefits for many men, it's essential to weigh the risks and tailor the treatment to each individual's needs. *Regular monitoring, including blood tests, cardiovascular assessments, and prostate health screenings, is critical to safely and effectively manage the therapy.* Careful consideration of all these factors ensures that TOT is administered in a way that maximizes benefits while minimizing potential risks.

The Role of Estrogen Blockers in Testosterone Optimization Therapy

In VitalLife, estrogen blockers play a vital role in hormone optimization for men undergoing testosterone therapy. While testosterone is the primary male hormone, a portion of it naturally converts into estrogen through a process called *aromatization*. A small amount of estrogen is important for maintaining various bodily functions, including bone health, but excessive estrogen in men can lead to unwanted side effects. These include water retention, gynecomastia (enlarged breast tissue), mood swings, and decreased libido. Estrogen blockers are prescribed to block the conversion of testosterone into estrogen, so that more testosterone is available, for better results. In VitalLife, estrogen blockers are almost always incorporated into testosterone optimization protocols.

There are two primary types of estrogen blockers used in men's hormone therapy: *aromatase inhibitors (AIs)* and *selective estrogen receptor modulators (SERMs)*. Aromatase inhibitors, such as anastrozole (Arimidex), letrozole (Femara), and exemestane (Aromasin), work by inhibiting the enzyme aromatase, which is responsible for converting testosterone into estrogen. This reduces overall estrogen levels in the body, helping prevent the side effects associated with elevated estrogen.

On the other hand, SERMs such as tamoxifen (Nolvadex) and clomiphene (Clomid) act by blocking estrogen receptors in specific tissues, particularly breast tissue, preventing estrogen from binding and causing gynecomastia or other related issues. SERMs are useful for targeting specific areas without significantly lowering overall estrogen levels, which can be important for maintaining optimal bone density and cardiovascular health.

Incorporating estrogen blockers along with certain peptides and even oxytocin (discussed later) into a comprehensive testosterone hormone optimization plan is essential to achieving the right hormonal balance, ensuring that testosterone levels are elevated while keeping estrogen within a healthy range. The key is finding the right balance—too much estrogen suppression can lead to side effects such as joint pain, fatigue, and an increased risk of bone loss, while too little can lead to estrogen dominance and its associated symptoms. That's why I obsess on monitoring biomarkers on regular basis and adjusting the treatment protocol as needed.

The HCG and Gonadorelin in Testosterone Optimization Treatment

Human chorionic gonadotropin (HCG) can play an important role in testosterone optimization therapy for men by maintaining testicular function during treatment. While exogenous testosterone can suppress the body's natural production of the hormone, HCG mimics luteinizing hormone (LH), stimulating the testes to produce testosterone and preserving fertility. This is particularly important for men who wish to maintain sperm production or prevent testicular atrophy while on therapy. In my experience, HCG not only complements testosterone optimization but also helps men sustain a more natural hormonal balance, supporting overall vitality and well-being.

Gonadorelin, a gonadotropin-releasing hormone (GnRH) analog, offers another effective approach in testosterone optimization therapy by stimulating the pituitary gland to release both luteinizing hormone (LH) and follicle-stimulating hormone (FSH). This action directly supports the testes in producing testosterone and sperm, making it an excellent choice for men concerned about fertility or the testicular shrinkage that can occur with TOT. Gonadorelin provides a more physiologic alternative to exogenous testosterone by encouraging the body's natural hormonal pathways. In my practice, I use it more often than HCG now. I've found it to be a valuable tool in personalized hormone optimization plans, ensuring men achieve their health and performance goals without compromising future reproductive potential.

Hormone Optimization Therapy (HOT) in Women: A Comprehensive Protocol

Let me share something I've observed from my medical experience working with women navigating their hormonal transitions. When your body begins its natural shift through perimenopause and menopause, it's not just a simple decline in estrogen—it's a sophisticated orchestration involving multiple hormonal systems. Also, these hormones function as vital messengers, influencing not just reproductive health, but your entire body's resilience and vitality. This intricate hormonal dance affects everything from cellular energy production to neurotransmitter balance. That's why when hormone levels shift, you might notice changes across multiple dimensions of your well-being.

I've come to see hormone optimization as an art as much as a science. Yes, what we're talking about is commonly referred to as hormone replacement therapy (HRT), but I prefer to think of it as *Hormone Optimization Therapy* (*HOT*), orchestrating your body's natural wisdom. When done with precision and deep understanding, *this approach doesn't just "replace" what's missing—it helps restore your entire hormonal ecosystem to its natural rhythm.*

Take *estrogen*, for example. It's one of the most important hormones in a woman's body, responsible for everything from maintaining bone density to regulating mood and keeping the skin healthy. When estrogen levels drop, women may start experiencing hot flashes, night sweats, vaginal dryness, and even changes in mood, such as feeling more anxious or irritable than usual. On top of that, many women report sleep disturbances, low energy, and even a sense of mental fogginess. What's often overlooked is the long-term impact of low estrogen, like an increased risk of osteoporosis and heart disease. That's why hormone replacement can be such a game changer.

When it comes to prescribing estrogen, there are several options available. Some women prefer oral tablets, which are easy to take, while others might opt for transdermal patches or gels that deliver estrogen directly through the skin with a lower risk of side effects like blood clots. For women struggling with vaginal symptoms, vaginal creams can be a great option to target dryness and discomfort without affecting the entire system. The key is finding the form of estrogen that fits your lifestyle and needs. And for those looking for a more natural approach, bioidentical hormones, which are chemically identical to the ones your body naturally produces, are becoming more popular. These are often derived from plants and can be tailored to suit your body's unique requirements.

But let's not forget about *progesterone*, which is just as important, especially if you still have your uterus. Unless she has gone through hysterectomy, taking estrogen without balancing it with progesterone can lead to the overgrowth of the uterine lining, which increases the risk of cancer. Progesterone helps to keep things in check and also has the added benefit of supporting better sleep, stabilizing mood, and even offering some neuroprotective effects. There are different forms of progesterone to choose from as well. *Micronized progesterone*, which is bioidentical, is a great option for women looking for fewer side effects, while *synthetic progestins* are available but can sometimes lead to issues like mood swings or breast tenderness. Finding the right balance between estrogen and progesterone is key to feeling your best.

Now, you might not think of *testosterone* as a hormone that's important for women, but it plays a huge role in women's sexual health, energy levels, and mental clarity. As testosterone levels drop with age, women may notice a decline in libido, muscle tone, and overall vitality. For some women, adding a small dose of testosterone can help reignite their sex drive, increase energy, and even improve mood. Testosterone therapy for women can be administered through creams, gels, or even pellets implanted under the skin for a steady release. However, it's important to monitor levels carefully, as too much testosterone can lead to unwanted side effects like acne or facial hair.

As we discussed earlier, hormone optimization in women requires more than simply replacing what's missing. By considering not just estrogen and progesterone but also testosterone and other bioidentical options, we can create a personalized plan that restores balance and supports long-term wellness. Add to that support for metabolism, gut health, and cellular energy production, and you've got a comprehensive approach to hormone optimization that can make a real difference in how women feel as they age. It's about taking control of the changes your body is going through and making choices that help you thrive.

Side Effects and Precautions of Hormone Treatments in Women

While hormone optimization can be highly effective for many women, it's important to recognize that it comes with potential risks and side effects. As with any treatment, hormone therapy needs to be carefully monitored and personalized. It's not for everyone, and certain women may face more risks than benefits.

Some common side effects of estrogen therapy include bloating, breast tenderness, mood swings, and headaches. In some women, there may be weight gain or fluid retention, especially in the early stages of therapy. Oral estrogen can increase the risk of blood clots, stroke, and heart attack, particularly in women with underlying risk factors like high blood pressure or a history of smoking. For this reason, transdermal options such as gels or patches are often recommended, as they are shown to carry a lower risk.

Using estrogen alone can make the inside lining of the uterus too thick—a disorder called estrogen-related endometrial hyperplasia. This raises your risk for cancer of the uterus. The progesterone combined with estrogen can prevent this from happening.

Another concern with long-term hormone therapy in women is the slight increase in the risk of breast cancer, especially when combining estrogen and progesterone, with the risk growing the longer it is taken. Women with a family history of breast cancer or other risk factors should carefully weigh the potential risks. Constant monitoring and physician oversight is the key to avoid serious complications.

Progesterone and progestin therapy side effects can include fatigue, mood changes, or spotting. Synthetic progestins can lead to more side effects, such as breast tenderness and fluid retention, which is why micronized bioidentical progesterone is often preferred—it has better tolerability.

Those with a history of breast cancer, endometrial cancer, blood clots, stroke, or heart disease are typically advised against HRT due to the potential risks. Women with severe liver disease, gallbladder disease, or uncontrolled high blood pressure should also avoid hormone therapy. Women who experience migraines with aura or have a history of migraines may need to be cautious with estrogen therapy, as it can worsen their symptoms.

The key to safe and effective HOT is regular monitoring with tests and physician oversight. Routine blood tests, mammograms, and pelvic exams are essential to ensure hormone levels are balanced and to catch any issues early. Women at risk for osteoporosis should also undergo bone density scans. Ultimately, while HOT can offer many benefits, it must be tailored to each woman's unique health profile, with regular assessments to ensure safety. It's about finding the right balance, addressing symptoms, and managing potential risks with a comprehensive approach.

More Hormones and Peptides in Comprehensive Hormone Optimization

In addition to the more commonly discussed hormones like testosterone, estrogen, and progesterone, the VitalLife program integrates a range of other hormones and peptides that play crucial roles in optimizing health, vitality, and longevity. While some of these therapies are more mainstream, others are used with caution due to their controversial nature, as well as potential risks and benefits. Let's dive into each of these in detail.

Growth Hormone: A Controversial Tool, Used Sparingly

Growth hormone (GH), or human growth hormone (HGH), is often associated with the body's growth and cellular regeneration. When used appropriately, GH can improve muscle mass, fat distribution, skin elasticity, and energy levels. It can also support bone density and wound healing. While it has significant benefits, it is also a controversial hormone, particularly when used in adults. In hormone optimization, growth hormone is used sparingly and only in carefully selected patients, often those with growth hormone deficiency or patients requiring enhanced cell regeneration or metabolic support.

Potential side effects can include joint pain, carpal tunnel syndrome, edema (fluid retention), and increased risk of insulin resistance. Long-term use or misuse or using it as performance enhancer can increase the risk of cardiovascular disease and potentially promote the growth of cancer cells, which is why GH therapy must be used cautiously and sparingly, with very strict monitoring.

Oxytocin: The Bonding Hormone

Oxytocin, often called the "love hormone" or "bonding hormone," plays a crucial role in social bonding, emotional well-being, and even sexual health. It is naturally released during intimacy, childbirth, and breastfeeding, but it can also be supplemented therapeutically. Oxytocin can be used to enhance emotional bonding, improve intimacy, and support overall emotional balance. In the context of hormone optimization, it may be used to promote a sense of well-being, reduce stress, and help restore relationships that have been affected by hormonal imbalance. Potential side effects are minimal but can include nausea, headaches, and mild irritability in some individuals.

Interestingly, studies have revealed that interactions with pets trigger the release of oxytocin too, which plays a key role in fostering health benefits such as reduced stress and improved emotional well-being. Research also suggests that pets, particularly dogs, possess the extraordinary ability to smell their owner's oxytocin levels and changes in their stress state, further deepening the bond and their role in supporting human health.

DHEA: The Anti-aging Hormone

DHEA (dehydroepiandrosterone) is a hormone produced by the adrenal glands that acts as a precursor to testosterone and estrogen. DHEA levels decline with age, and supplementation is often used to support energy levels, immune function, and hormonal balance. DHEA is often used as part of anti-aging protocols to restore youthful hormone levels and support metabolism and muscle maintenance.

DHEA can help with fat loss, increased energy, improved mood, and even sexual function. It also has a role in supporting the immune system and maintaining bone density. Excess DHEA can lead to acne, hair loss, oily skin, and, in some cases, irritability. In women, too much DHEA may cause facial hair growth and voice deepening. Long-term use may also affect cholesterol levels.

Thyroid Hormones: The Metabolic Regulators

Thyroid hormones, including T3 (triiodothyronine) and T4 (thyroxine), are essential for regulating metabolism, energy production, and overall body function. As women and men age, thyroid function can decline, leading to hypothyroidism (underactive thyroid), which can cause weight gain, fatigue, depression, and cold intolerance.

Thyroid hormone replacement therapy is used to bring hormone levels back into balance, optimizing metabolism, energy levels, and mental clarity. Treatment usually involves synthetic or bioidentical forms of T3 and T4. Thyroid hormone therapy can significantly improve energy levels, mental focus, weight management, and mood stability. Over-replacement can cause hyperthyroid-like symptoms, including heart palpitations, anxiety, insomnia, and osteoporosis over time. Regular monitoring is crucial to avoid these risks.

Melatonin: Sleep and Beyond

Melatonin is a hormone naturally produced by the pineal gland that regulates the sleep-wake cycle. While primarily known as a sleep aid, melatonin has antioxidant properties and plays a role in immune function, anti-aging, and even cancer prevention. Melatonin is used primarily to regulate sleep patterns, but I have also used it for its broader benefits, such as immune support and anti-inflammatory effects.

Melatonin supplementation improves sleep quality, regulates circadian rhythms, and may support cognitive health. It can also be beneficial in protecting against oxidative stress and age-related decline. Melatonin is generally safe, though in some cases, it may cause drowsiness during the day, headaches, or vivid dreams.

Pregnenolone: The Memory Hormone

Pregnenolone is another adrenal hormone that serves as a precursor to other hormones, including progesterone, DHEA, and estrogen. Known as the "memory hormone," pregnenolone is linked to cognitive function, memory retention, and mood stabilization. Pregnenolone is often used orally to support brain function, particularly in aging individuals, and to balance other hormones in the body.

It may enhance memory, reduce stress, and improve mood, particularly in those experiencing cognitive decline or mood disorders related to aging. Excess pregnenolone can lead to anxiety, insomnia, or irritability. It can also impact the balance of other hormones, so close monitoring is important.

Peptides Optimization

Peptides like sermorelin or PT-141 are also used in VitalLife. These therapies focus on improving cell regeneration, muscle mass, and sexual function.

- **Sermorelin:** It stimulates the pituitary gland to produce *natural growth hormone*, thus aiding in muscle recovery, sleep, and metabolism without the risks associated with direct GH therapy. It's commonly used to support muscle growth, improve sleep, boost energy, and promote cellular repair. Since sermorelin works with the body's own systems, *it tends to carry fewer risks than synthetic growth hormone*, making it a safer option for enhancing vitality and overall health. This can be administered as injectable or a rapid-dissolve oral tablet.
- **PT-141:** Also known as *Bremelanotide*, is a peptide used primarily to enhance sexual function in both men and women. Unlike traditional treatments for sexual dysfunction, which work by increasing blood flow, PT-141 acts on the nervous system by stimulating receptors in the brain related to desire. It is commonly used to treat ED, low libido, and sexual arousal disorders, improving sexual desire and performance. PT-141 is typically administered via oral or subcutaneous injection, and while generally well tolerated, some potential side effects include nausea, flushing, and headaches.
- **BPC-157 (*Wolverine peptide*):** It is a synthetic peptide derived from a protein found in the stomach, and it's known for its powerful healing properties. It promotes the repair of tissues, especially in the muscles, tendons, and ligaments, making it popular in the treatment of injuries and inflammatory conditions. BPC-157 has also been shown to support gut health, aiding in the healing of the gastrointestinal lining. It is typically administered via

injection, and while generally considered safe, it is still under study, with potential side effects and long-term safety not yet fully established.

—

As we bring this discussion to a close, we've seen how a proper and comprehensive hormone optimization through balancing multiple hormones and peptides is vital to reclaiming energy, youthfulness, and well-being. Each of these therapies works together to help you feel more like yourself again. But of course, it's all about finding the right balance, fine-tuning, continuous monitoring, adjusting where needed, and being mindful of the risks and benefits that come with hormone therapy.

It is so crucial to recognize that even the best hormone and peptide optimization does not function in isolation. Based on your specific medical needs and biomarker results, hormone and peptide therapy should be combined with additional modalities to maximize results. This means taking a holistic view of your health, encompassing the entire VitalLife program, which embraces so many years of clinical experience.

Now that we've tackled the role of hormones and peptides, let's shift focus to another crucial area—metabolism and insulin resistance. In the next chapter, we'll explore how mastering your metabolism and addressing insulin resistance can unlock a whole new level of health and energy for years to come.

CHAPTER 12

Mastering Metabolism: Mitochondrial Dysfunction and Insulin Resistance

A man who loves to walk will walk farther than a man who loves the destination.
—Attributed to Lao-tzu, Chinese philosopher of the sixth century BC

Everybody needs a hug. It changes your metabolism.
—Leo Buscaglia, American author and motivational speaker (1924–1998)

Let me share the story of another one of my patients, Joshua, a professional NFL player, who came to me at the age of thirty-two. He was at a point where his energy was declining, his focus was off, and he was struggling with weight gain and poor sleep. Despite his best efforts on the field, he felt like his body wasn't keeping up with the demands of his sport, and it was starting to affect his performance and overall well-being. As an athlete used to pushing himself to excel, Joshua was frustrated, with his confidence hitting rock bottom. He knew he needed a real solution.

In designing a customized program for him, I took a comprehensive approach, addressing every aspect of his health. After a thorough biomarker assessment including a robust peak athletic performance testing, I designed a personalized plan for him. By optimizing his peptides (without any hormones) and cellular metabolism, incorporating an anti-inflammatory diet, a tailored supplement regimen, a few compounded IV therapies, and using select localized regenerative therapies to help his body repair itself, Joshua began to see significant changes. Within three months, he regained his youthful energy and stamina. His sleep improved, his focus sharpened, and he lost weight—all the while building lean muscle mass and strength. His performance on the field improved, but more importantly, he felt like himself again—stronger, more resilient and confident, and ready to take on the challenges ahead.

Joshua's story is just one example of how a comprehensive and personalized approach can create real, lasting change. Whether you're an elite athlete or someone simply wanting to feel better and live a more vibrant life, VitalLife program offers the tools to restore your health and help you thrive. With the right combination of regenerative medicine, personalized treatments, and lifestyle changes, Joshua's transformation proves that a healthier, more vibrant version of yourself is within reach.

Insulin Resistance and Role of the Mitochondria

At the core of my experience in anti-aging lies a crucial truth of the Aging Triad that we discussed in chapter 6: chronic inflammation, metabolism insulin resistance, and mitochondrial dysfunction figure prominently in determining how well our bodies age. Metabolism governs the process by which cells convert nutrients into usable energy, fueling everything from muscle contraction to brain function. Science is clear: a consistently diminished mitochondrial function and metabolic efficiency leads to reduced energy levels, diminished physical performance, and impaired tissue repair.

As we discussed in chapter 5—and it is worth reviewing briefly here—*metabolic health is essentially about insulin resistance and mitochondrial dysfunction lies at the heart of insulin resistance, caused by environmental toxins, unhealthy fats, ultra-processed food, gut dysbiosis, and an excessive calorie workload* on these cellular powerhouses from simply eating too many calories in our Western diet. When mitochondria are damaged, cell receptors fail to allow sugar into cells, leaving high levels of sugar in the bloodstream despite sufficient insulin. This is the essence of insulin resistance when cells simply can't hear insulin's signals, a condition that serves as the gateway to a cascade of complications. *The key point here is that the high sugar is more of a symptom; the root cause lies in the Aging Triad. This is why addressing the underlying factors of Aging Triad is critical for restoring metabolic health and reversing diseases.*

Over the years, thousands of studies have been published on the *relationship between diet, metabolic health, and diseases*—particularly heart disease, obesity, and diabetes. Let me share a few key findings that highlight important concepts in insulin resistance.

In 1927 a study published in the *Archives of Internal Medicine* evaluated the effects of two types of diets on insulin resistance in young, healthy volunteers. Researchers studied medical students in their twenties, dividing them into two groups. One group consumed a fat-rich diet, including bacon, eggs, cream, butter, and oils. The other group followed a carb-rich diet consisting of sugar, pastries, candy, white bread, rice, potatoes, oatmeal, and syrup. Guess who showed more insulin resistance within a few days with an increase in blood sugar levels? It was the group that received the fat-rich diet.

Fast forward to 2008, when a study published in the *New England Journal of Medicine* found that intensive blood sugar control in diabetic patients actually increased mortality rates. The results were so concerning that researchers had to stop the study early for safety reasons.

Study after study confirm what we discussed in chapters 5 and 6—*it's the fat, not the sugar*, in our diet that disrupts cellular and mitochondrial function, leading to insulin resistance. Sugar in one's diet may elevate blood sugar levels, but it's not the root cause of insulin resistance. The real culprit is fat, and not just saturated or trans fats, but all kinds of fats.

The reverse is also true. Reducing fat in the bloodstream improves insulin resistance. For example, a 2009 study published in the *Journal of Clinical Nutrition* showed that switching to a vegetarian diet (including dairy and eggs) reduced the prevalence of diabetes by 61 percent. Even more impressive, switching to a completely plant-based diet—with no meat, dairy, or eggs—reduced diabetes prevalence by nearly 80 percent.

Here's the best part: it's never too late to start making changes to reverse disease and optimize your health. Multiple clinical studies led by many pioneers, such as Nathan Pritikin, Dr. Dean Ornish, and Dr. Caldwell Esselstyn Jr. among others, have clearly demonstrated, utilizing objective data from coronary angiograms (a dye test to examine the blood vessels of the heart), that *even the progression of severe coronary heart disease—often necessitating surgery—can be reversed by making comprehensive changes in diet and lifestyle.*

The takeaway is simple: if you provide your body with the right conditions, it has an incredible ability to heal itself. In that sense, *insulin resistance, diabetes, heart disease, and stroke are all diseases of choice—PREVENTABLE and REVERSIBLE with the right lifestyle changes and health strategies.* In the VitalLife program, I've developed specific protocols that restore insulin sensitivity, effectively managing metabolic health and slowing the aging process. I'm passionate about this because this helps us in achieving our goal of not just extending lifespan, but also maximizing healthspan, ensuring our future years are lived with vibrancy, strength, and optimal health.

Practical Strategies to Combat Mitochondrial Dysfunction and Insulin Resistance

Let's delve into practical strategies that have consistently delivered remarkable results in restoring metabolic health. I have witnessed these interventions transform lives when carefully tailored to an individual's medical history, biomarkers, and unique health goals.

First Step: Detoxification

The very first key step in supporting mitochondrial function is detoxifying the body, starting with avoiding the *"unholy trinity"* of smoking, drinking alcohol, and poor foods, as we will discuss in detail in chapter 15, where we delve into nutrition. The cornerstone of metabolic mastery begins with dietary intervention. The profound impact of what we eat on insulin regulation, mitochondrial function, and energy processing cannot be overstated. Research has shown that diets high in processed and fried foods are strongly correlated with increased rates of type 2 diabetes and metabolic syndrome. *We need to begin by removing unhealthy fats, ultra-processed food, fried foods, and calorie-dense items form our diets.*

Additionally, minimizing exposure to endocrine disruptors is crucial. Environmental toxins like bisphenol A (BPA), phthalates, hormones, and pesticides can disrupt hormonal balance and impair insulin function. You can reduce these harmful effects with few simple steps, including opting for glass or stainless-steel containers, steering clear of processed and refined foods, and choosing organic produce whenever possible.

The Foundation: Nutrition as a Catalyst for Change

I have devoted an entire chapter, chapter 15, to this topic. Nutrition is not just a meal plan—it's a powerful tool for reclaiming metabolic and overall health. Let us discuss a few of these nutritional strategies specific to our metabolism. The solution lies in transforming your nutritional landscape. *Prioritize whole, nutrient-dense foods* such as dark leafy greens, cruciferous vegetables, plant-based proteins, healthy fats from sources like avocados and nuts, legumes, and fiber-rich grains such as quinoa or oats. These foods promote steady insulin release and enhance overall sensitivity.

Foods high in antioxidant compounds called polyphenols, such as *green tea, dark chocolate, berries, and red wine* (in small amounts), have been shown to reduce oxidative stress and improve glucose uptake by enhancing GLUT4 receptor activity. Green tea, specifically, contains catechins that enhance fat oxidation and insulin sensitivity. *Advanced glycation end products*, or AGEs, are harmful compounds formed when proteins or fats combine with sugar during cooking, especially at high temperatures. Limiting foods cooked at high heat (for example, fried or smoked) and opting for light grilling, baking, steaming, or boiling can reduce AGEs and might improve insulin sensitivity. Other foods that are high in AGEs and need to be avoided include red meat, high-fructose corn syrup, ultra-processed foods, certain cheeses, cream cheese, margarine, and mayonnaise.

Intermittent fasting and time-restricted eating have been shown to improve insulin sensitivity by reducing fasting insulin levels and allowing cells to reset their metabolic processes. Studies suggest that fasting periods of twelve to sixteen hours can enhance mitochondrial function, reduce inflammation, and improve glucose metabolism.

Note: For all my patients, *I target for a total cholesterol level less than 150 mg/dl and an LDL (bad cholesterol) level under 70 mg/dl.* It is a more aggressive approach than recommended by the American Heart Association. And this is possible to achieve with a strict plant-based diet, even without any medications.

Gut Microbiome

The gut microbiome plays a pivotal role in metabolic health. Imbalances in gut bacteria (dysbiosis) are linked to insulin resistance and systemic inflammation. As we'll discuss in detail in the next chapter, strategies like increasing dietary fiber, consuming fermented foods (for example, yogurt, kefir, sauerkraut), and taking targeted probiotics and herbs can restore microbiome balance, improving insulin sensitivity.

Advanced Natural Compounds: The Metabolism Helpers

Certain compounds and supplements have demonstrated remarkable potential in supporting your metabolic health. *Alpha-lipoic acid (ALA)*, a powerful antioxidant, supports mitochondrial function while reducing oxidative stress linked to insulin resistance. *Magnesium* is essential for more than three hundred enzymatic reactions, many of which involve glucose metabolism. *Berberine*, often compared to the drug metformin, has been shown in studies to enhance glucose metabolism and reduce insulin resistance, making it a favorite as a natural medicine. *Chromium* improves carbohydrate metabolism, while *vitamin D_3* plays a crucial role in regulating insulin and glucose homeostasis, with deficiencies linked to metabolic disorders. *Omega-3 fatty acids* and *coenzyme Q10 (CoQ10)* further protect against inflammation and oxidative damage, providing essential support for mitochondrial health and metabolic function.

For those seeking comprehensive metabolic support, I find that compounds like resveratrol, N-acetylcysteine (NAC), and quercetin offer synergistic benefits. *Resveratrol*, a compound found in red wine and berries, activates pathways that enhance insulin sensitivity and mitochondrial function. *NAC* supports glutathione production, protecting cells from oxidative stress, while *quercetin* reduces inflammation and improves glucose metabolism.

Mitopure, a highly purified form of *urolithin A*, has emerged as a groundbreaking compound for improving mitochondrial function. Urolithin A, a natural compound found in pomegranates, walnuts, almonds, and strawberries, works by enhancing *mitophagy*, a process by which damaged mitochondria are identified and removed, making way for healthier, more efficient mitochondria. Studies have shown that Mitopure boosts cellular energy production, reduces oxidative stress, and improves muscle strength and endurance, particularly in aging individuals. By targeting mitochondrial health at its core, Mitopure offers a promising solution for promoting vitality, longevity, and overall cellular function.

Pyrroloquinoline quinone (*PQQ*) is a potent antioxidant and cofactor that supports mitochondrial health and function. It stimulates the growth of new mitochondria—a process known as mitochondrial biogenesis—while protecting existing mitochondria from oxidative damage. PQQ has been shown to improve cellular energy production, enhance brain function, and reduce inflammation, making it particularly valuable for combating age-related declines in mitochondrial efficiency. By revitalizing the "powerhouses" of the cell, PQQ plays a critical role in promoting energy, longevity, and overall health.

These interventions work hand in hand with lifestyle modifications and foundational therapies to address metabolic dysfunction holistically. They offer additional layers of protection and optimization for those striving to achieve long-term health and vitality.

Exercise: A Cornerstone of Metabolic Health

Studies consistently show that even moderate exercise can improve insulin sensitivity and reduce abdominal fat, a significant contributor to metabolic dysfunction. Regular physical activity also boosts mitochondrial function, allowing cells to produce energy more efficiently. Movement is more than exercise; it's a daily investment in long-term vitality. Both aerobic and strength training improve insulin sensitivity by increasing glucose uptake in muscles. High-intensity interval training (HIIT), which alternates between short bursts of intense exercise and rest, has been shown to extend insulin sensitivity for hours after a workout. Resistance training, particularly as we age, is vital for preserving muscle mass—a key determinant of metabolic health—while also enhancing glucose utilization.

Stress Management and Restful Sleep: The Silent Influencers

Stress is often overlooked in discussions about metabolic health, but its impact is profound. Chronic stress elevates cortisol levels, which in turn promotes insulin resistance and visceral fat accumulation, particularly around the abdomen. Over time, this hormonal disruption fuels systemic inflammation and impairs metabolic balance.

Mindfulness practices such as meditation, yoga, and deep breathing exercises can lower your cortisol levels and support metabolic health. Research highlights the direct link between stress reduction and improved insulin sensitivity. Incorporating these practices into daily routines provides a powerful, non-pharmacological way to break the cycle of stress-induced metabolic dysfunction.

Chronic sleep deprivation is strongly associated with insulin resistance. Improving your sleep quality through consistent sleep schedules, minimizing blue light exposure before bed, and optimizing sleep environments can significantly enhance metabolic health. Research has shown that even one week of poor sleep can reduce insulin sensitivity by up to 30 percent.

Metabolic Medications: Evidence-Based Support

For enhanced metabolic management, certain medications have shown significant benefits. *Metformin*, widely used for type 2 diabetes, improves insulin sensitivity and lowers glucose production in the liver. It is also gaining attention in longevity research for its potential anti-aging effects. *Thiazolidinediones (TZDs)*, such as pioglitazone, enhance glucose uptake in adipose tissue, while *GLP-1 agonists* like semaglutide and liraglutide optimize insulin secretion and reduce appetite. These medications, when used appropriately, can complement lifestyle interventions. However, the key lies in understanding that medications work best when paired with foundational changes in nutrition, movement, and stress management.

Traditional Herbal Medicine: Timeless Remedies for Optimal Metabolism

The wisdom of traditional medicine offers additional tools for managing metabolic health. *Fenugreek*, rich in soluble fiber, supports balanced blood sugar and improves insulin sensitivity. *Bitter melon* contains natural compounds that mimic insulin's effects, enhancing glucose uptake. *American ginseng* has demonstrated significant benefits in improving glucose control, while *turmeric*, with its active compound curcumin, exhibits potent anti-inflammatory properties that improve insulin sensitivity. Similarly, *cinnamon* helps regulate blood sugar levels by enhancing glucose uptake in cells.

Holy basil, a revered herb in Ayurvedic medicine, shows potential in regulating blood sugar and supporting overall metabolic health. These natural remedies, backed by emerging science, complement modern approaches, bridging the gap between tradition and innovation.

A simple recipe I recommend to my patients, particularly those with obesity and insulin resistance, is to *combine lemon, ginger, turmeric, and green tea leaves*, adding small amounts of honey as needed. This can be consumed three to four times a day to help boost metabolism and reduce inflammation in the body.

Cold Exposure and Thermogenesis

Exposure to cold temperatures has a powerful effect on your body's metabolism, primarily by *activating brown adipose tissue (BAT)*. Unlike white fat, which stores energy, BAT burns glucose and fatty acids to generate heat in a process called thermogenesis. This activation not only helps the body maintain temperature but also significantly improves insulin sensitivity and glucose metabolism, making it a promising tool for managing metabolic health.

Techniques such as cold showers, ice baths, and advanced cryotherapy chambers are gaining popularity for their ability to harness these effects. Studies suggest that regular cold exposure can increase calorie burn, improve lipid profiles, and support overall metabolic function, offering a natural and accessible way to optimize health.

Advanced Peptides

Peptides have emerged as powerful tools in improving mitochondrial function and combating insulin resistance, offering targeted and effective interventions for metabolic health. BPC-157, known as the "body-protecting compound," is highly effective in reducing inflammation and promoting cellular repair. By supporting mitochondrial health and reducing oxidative stress, BPC-157 enhances the ability of cells to utilize energy efficiently, making it a valuable ally in addressing metabolic dysfunction.

Two other standout peptides are *sermorelin* and *tesamorelin*, which stimulate the release of growth hormone and have shown significant benefits in reducing visceral fat in a select patient population. By decreasing abdominal fat—a major contributor to insulin resistance—they help improve glucose metabolism and insulin sensitivity. However, be cautious, as in some patients, these can actually raise blood sugar levels and exacerbate diabetes. Similarly, *CJC-1295* and *ipamorelin* (a synthetic hormone ghrelin analog), when used together, boost growth hormone secretion, supporting mitochondrial biogenesis and overall metabolic function. These peptides play a crucial role in preserving muscle mass, enhancing fat utilization, and promoting healthy aging. Some people can see their blood sugar levels rise.

For individuals with severe insulin resistance or mitochondrial dysfunction, a naturally occurring peptide found in thymus gland, *thymosin alpha 1*, can also be helpful. It modulates immune function, reducing chronic inflammation—a key driver of mitochondrial damage and insulin resistance. In addition, *Semax*, a neuropeptide approved in a few European countries but not in the United States, supports oxidative stress reduction and improves cellular energy production, indirectly enhancing metabolic function.

Some of these peptides have shown promise in laboratory settings so far, and I mention them here to monitor their potential for the near future. AOD9604, originally developed as an anti-obesity peptide, has demonstrated potential in improving fat metabolism and supporting mitochondrial function. By mimicking the fat-burning action of growth hormone without affecting glucose levels, it offers a unique approach to tackling insulin resistance. *MOTS-c*, an experimental peptide encoded in mitochondrial DNA, is not legally available for human consumption. It can directly improve mitochondrial function by enhancing glucose uptake and reducing insulin resistance at the cellular level. Its ability to mimic the effects of exercise on mitochondrial health has made it a focus of cutting-edge metabolic research.

Collectively, these peptides work *synergistically* to address the root causes of metabolic dysfunction, supporting mitochondrial health, reducing inflammation, and improving insulin sensitivity. As part of a personalized treatment plan, they offer a cutting-edge approach to restoring balance and vitality in metabolic health.

Specific Strategies to Curb Sarcopenia

As we discussed in chapter 6, sarcopenia refers to the loss of both muscle size and strength. *Evidence suggests that this decline starts as early as in your forties* and continues downward in a linear fashion. In my clinical experience, I've seen how sarcopenia profoundly impacts people's lives, particularly in their sixties and beyond, leaving them frail, less mobile, and more vulnerable to falls and fractures.

> Sarcopenia might be the common disease you never heard of. Research shows the importance of targeting sarcopenia as an important part of maintaining youthfulness and longevity.

It is a key contributor to the aging process, making prevention and treatment essential components of any longevity program. Addressing sarcopenia is a crucial part of VitalLife, with detailed treatments outlined below. If left unchecked, sarcopenia can progress quickly, *especially in people with chronic diseases like diabetes, heart dis-*

ease, or *cancer*, which are already linked to muscle loss. But here's the good news: I've seen firsthand how these strategies discussed below can significantly slow down or even reverse sarcopenia.

By addressing its root causes through a multifaceted approach, we can effectively rebuild muscle mass, restore strength, and enhance overall vitality. Here are the most impactful interventions for treating sarcopenia, incorporating the latest research and practical applications.

Resistance Training: The Cornerstone of Muscle Health

As we will discuss in detail in chapter 16, resistance training is the single most effective intervention for reversing sarcopenia. Exercises such as weightlifting, resistance band workouts, and bodyweight training stimulate muscle protein synthesis and increase muscle strength. Regular sessions, tailored to individual capacity and gradually intensified, not only help rebuild muscle but also improve balance, endurance, and overall functionality.

Optimizing Protein Intake

Adequate dietary protein is essential for muscle maintenance and repair. Aiming for 1 to 1.5 grams of protein per kilogram of body weight daily is ideal for supporting muscle synthesis in most healthy people. High-quality protein sources, such as peas, hemp, chia, almonds, and *sacha inchi*, should be prioritized.

L-Leucine and HMB

L-leucine, a branched-chain amino acid (BCAA), plays a critical role in activating muscle protein synthesis. Its metabolite, beta-hydroxy-beta-methyl butyrate (HMB), has been shown to preserve muscle mass, especially in older adults. Including these amino acids as part of a supplement regimen can significantly enhance muscle repair and growth.

Hormone Optimization

Hormonal imbalances are a major driver of sarcopenia. As we discussed in earlier chapters, optimizing levels of testosterone, growth hormone, and insulin-like growth factor-1 (IGF-1) is crucial. Treatments that include hormones, peptides, and targeted pharmacy products can restore anabolic hormone levels, supporting muscle regeneration.

NAD+ and Cellular Support

NAD+ supplementation, a key player in mitochondrial health, helps improve cellular energy production, supporting muscle repair and recovery. NAD+ boosters are a foundational part of sarcopenia treatment.

Vitamins and Nutritional Supplements

Micronutrient deficiencies can exacerbate muscle loss. Specific vitamins and minerals such as vitamin D_3, omega-3 fatty acids, magnesium, and chromium have been shown to support muscle strength and reduce inflammation. Ensuring adequate levels of these nutrients is a critical aspect of any sarcopenia treatment plan.

Gut-Muscle Axis and Fiber-Rich Nutrition

Emerging research highlights the gut-muscle axis—a bidirectional relationship between gut health and muscle function. Increasing dietary fiber and incorporating prebiotics and probiotics can improve gut health, reduce systemic inflammation, and indirectly support muscle health. This approach underscores the importance of a healthy microbiome in any longevity program.

Research-Backed Compounds for Muscle Function

Several compounds have demonstrated significant benefits in improving muscle mass and function:

- **Creatine:** Enhances energy production in muscles, improving strength and endurance.
- **Amylopectin:** A highly branched polysaccharide, it is shown to support muscle recovery and regeneration.
- **HMB**: It helps improve lean muscle, strength, and function. It can also help with athletic performance and recovery.
- **Ursolic Acid:** Found in apple peels, this compound promotes muscle growth and reduces fat accumulation.
- **Urolithin A:** Discussed above, it has been shown to enhance mitochondrial function and improve muscle health, making it a promising addition to strategies aimed at combating sarcopenia and slowing age-related muscle decline.

By integrating these strategies into a personalized plan, one can not only manage, but reverse sarcopenia. Through resistance training, dietary adjustments, targeted supplements, and cutting-edge therapies, you can regain your strength, vitality, and the confidence to live fully at any age.

As we have discussed in this chapter, mastering metabolism is about taking control of the body's natural processes. By maintaining insulin sensitivity and optimizing metabolic function, you unlock the key to not only a longer life, but a life filled with energy, health, and vitality. So, you see that the secret to eternal youth wasn't a mythical quest, but a tangible reality within our grasp. By understanding and harnessing the power of proper cellular metabolism, we could unlock the door to a longer, healthier, and more vibrant life.

We have seen how our internal systems are intricately connected. Just as insulin sensitivity governs how efficiently our bodies process energy, the strength of our immune system plays a vital role in protecting our health and enhancing longevity. In the next chapter, we'll delve into how a well-functioning immune system is essential not only for defending against illness but also for promoting optimal health, youthfulness, reducing inflammation, and ensuring long-term vitality. By optimizing both metabolism and immunity, you create a powerful synergy that keeps your body resilient and thriving at every stage of life.

CHAPTER 13

Fighting Systemic Chronic Inflammation: Boosting Immune and Gut Health

> To get back my youth, I would do anything in the world, except take exercise, get up early, or be respectable.
> —Oscar Wilde, Irish writer (1854–1900)

> All disease begins in the gut.
> —Hippocrates, ancient Greek physician known as "Father of Medicine" (ca. 460 BC–ca. 370 BC)

Susan, a forty-five-year-old senior marketing executive, walked into my office looking utterly defeated. For years, she had been struggling under the weight of a cascade of symptoms that had robbed her of joy and vitality. She was overweight, plagued by joint stiffness and diffuse muscle aches, and constantly battling fatigue so profound that even getting through the day felt insurmountable. Her nights were no better—insomnia left her exhausted, and brain fog clouded her days. She spoke of feeling breathless after even a short walk, her stomach was perpetually bloated, and irritable bowel syndrome had become a regular source of discomfort. These relentless medical issues had pushed her into a deep depression, and poor sleep only magnified her misery. She had lost all interest in her family and her work.

When Susan sat across from me, she looked restless, anxious, and drained, her sadness palpable. There was no light in her eyes, no smile on her face. "I've lost my sunshine," she told me, her voice trembling with despair. Despite her diligent efforts—regular visits to her primary care physician and consultations with a slew of specialists, including a pain doctor, endocrinologist, gastroenterologist, psychiatrist, and cardiologist—she felt no better. She had a cabinet full of medications: pain relievers, pills for anxiety and depression, treatments for irritable bowel syndrome, Ozempic for weight loss, and even modafinil prescribed by her neurologist to combat fatigue and brain fog. Yet none of these provided meaningful relief. Worse still, at such a young age she had started to believe that she was beyond help.

I spent almost three hours with Susan that day, listening carefully to her story, examining her in detail, and meticulously reviewing the stack of lab reports, medical records, and medication bottles she had brought with her. Physically, aside from being overweight and visibly depressed, there were no clear signs of any specific disease. My initial impression was that her struggles might stem from an underlying autoimmune condition triggered by gut dysbiosis, likely provoked by poor diet and chronic stress—a possibility her numerous specialists had overlooked.

After undergoing thorough biomarker and biological tests, Susan embarked on a customized chronic inflammation protocol. This included a comprehensive detox regimen, microbiome protocol to combat gut dysbiosis, personalized compounded medications, carefully selected supplements, herbs, and—most importantly—lifestyle modifications centered around a gluten-free, plant-based diet with no processed foods. Two months later, when Susan returned to my office for another follow-up visit, she was almost unrecognizable. Her joint pain and muscle aches had eased, she was sleeping better, and her depression had significantly lifted. She had weaned off all the medications her specialists had prescribed, and for the first time in years, she felt a renewed sense of control over her life. The most rewarding moment for me was seeing her smile again—a smile filled with joy and confidence. "I finally feel like myself," she said, her voice brimming with hope.

Susan's story is far from unique. Over the years, I've treated countless patients who, like her, are burdened with multiple symptoms and shuffled between specialists. Too often, they are prescribed medications that only address the symptoms rather than the root cause. Worse still, these drugs frequently come with significant side effects, sometimes more debilitating than the original issues. Susan's journey is a reminder that when we look beyond the symptoms and focus on the root causes, true healing becomes possible.

Systemic Chronic Inflammation (SCI)

The intricate relationship between your immune system, systemic (meaning in your entire body) chronic inflammation, and aging reveals one of medicine's most fascinating frontiers. Through my years of experience as a physician—and through my own personal health challenges—I've developed not just an understanding, but a deep appreciation of how this low-grade, persistent inflammation can wreak havoc on every single cell and tissue in your body. As we have discussed earlier, particularly in chapter 5 where we explored the science of aging, *chronic inflammation has profoundly detrimental effects on our health.* I feel compelled to revisit this topic briefly here, for I deeply believe in its critical significance.

I believe systemic chronic inflammation represents one of medicine's most fascinating paradoxes—our own defense mechanisms can unintentionally harm the very tissues they are meant to protect. What's particularly striking is how an overactive immune response fuels this low-grade inflammation, often referred to as the "silent fire." This process revolves around the persistent production of pro-inflammatory cytokines, which keep the immune system in a constant state of alert. Over time, this accelerates aging and drives serious conditions such as atherosclerosis (arterial blockages), cardiovascular disease, type 2 diabetes, and cancer. Understanding and addressing this "silent fire" is essential for achieving optimal health and longevity.

> While aging is multifactorial, I believe this "silent fire" of chronic, low-grade inflammation in the entire body might be the MOST crucial factor determining your biological age, healthspan, and lifespan.

Interplay of Multiple Factors

What emerges from this understanding is that *your immune system is far more than just a defense against pathogens—it acts as a central orchestrator of the aging process.* Chronic inflammation impacts insulin sensitivity, causing a harmful cycle of high blood sugar and more inflammation. Combined with metabolic issues and abdominal fat, this cycle worsens, leading to chronic disease.

The immune system also manages "zombie" cells—senescent cells that harm tissues. Ideally, autophagy clears them, but with age, they accumulate, releasing harmful chemicals and accelerating aging. The gut microbiome is vital in immune responses and chronic inflammation. Modern research supports what Ayurveda has known: the gut, or "second brain," is linked to immune health. A balanced microbiome supports healthy immune responses, while an imbalanced one leads to leaky gut syndrome, systemic inflammation, and aging-related diseases. Epigenetics adds another layer. Chronic inflammation accelerates harmful epigenetic changes, degrading healthy cells and tissues, driving premature aging.

The Role of the Thymus Gland in Aging

The thymus is a small gland tucked behind the breastbone. It plays a critical role in our immune system, especially in our early years. However, as we age, the thymus undergoes a process called *thymic involution*—essentially shrinking and losing its function. By the time most of us reach our sixties, the thymus is often a shadow of its former self, significantly reducing the production of new immune cells. This decline contributes to the gradual weakening of the immune system over time. This loss of thymic function manifests in patients in various ways. It's not just about increased vulnerability to infections; it's also linked to chronic inflammation, autoimmune conditions, and even a higher risk of cancer.

Strategies to Counter Systemic Chronic Inflammation (SCI)

The path to preserving vitality and promoting healthy aging clearly begins with optimizing immune function. I've witnessed how, when properly supported, the immune system becomes a powerful ally in maintaining youthfulness, health, and longevity for years to come. Emerging strategies offer promising ways to counter and reverse immune function decline.

As a physician focused on longevity and optimizing healthspan, I want to share with you effective strategies for combating this systemic chronic inflammation that I've successfully implemented for my own health as well as the health of my family members and my patients in my practice.

Before starting any treatment protocol, I always begin with comprehensive baseline biomarker and biological age tests. Specifically for chronic inflammation, I utilize the specialized tests detailed in chapter 7, including white cell count, C3 and C4 complements, hs-CRP, ferritin, fibrinogen, ESR, Lp-PLA2, TNF-alpha, ESR, GlycA, and IL-6. For certain medical conditions, specific tests can be checked, such as rheumatoid factor, anti-DS DNA, and antinuclear antibody. *These tests not only provide valuable insights at the outset but are also repeated during the course of treatment to monitor progress, safeguard against complications, and adjust the protocol as needed.*

As I prescribe in my VitalLife program, with strategies listed below, you can actively combat the effects of chronic inflammation, protect against disease, and live a longer, energetic life.

Anti-inflammatory Diet

Let me start with what I consider the foundation: an anti-inflammatory diet. Clinical research has proved that chronic inflammation can be made worse—and better—with diet. In chapter 15, where we discuss nutrition, we'll explore this in detail. The core principle, however, lies in prioritizing *whole, nutrient-dense, plant-based foods while avoiding processed foods and environmental toxins such as hormones, pesticides, and preservatives.*

A study published in the *Journal of the American College of Cardiology* in 2020 followed, over time, a total of 210,145 individuals in the United States and assessed their diets from 1984 to 2016. Besides dietary habits, they also followed detailed inflammation biomarkers, and incidence of cardiovascular diseases (CVD), coronary heart disease (CHD), and stroke. What they found was that a diet high in red meat, processed meat, organ meat, refined carbohydrates, and sweetened beverages (*essentially the typical American diet*) was associated with elevated inflammation markers and a higher incidence of total CVD, CHD, and stroke. Consumption of this pro-inflammatory diet was clearly associated with a higher level of systemic, vascular, and metabolic inflammation and an unfavorable lipid profile. Individuals on this pro-inflammation diet had a 38 percent higher risk of developing CVD compared with people who followed a low-inflammation diet of green leafy vegetables, whole grain, fruits, and tea.

I've clinically observed remarkable improvements in patients who avoid all processed foods and incorporate abundant fruits and vegetables, rich in antioxidants and polyphenols that fight oxidative stress. I particularly emphasize foods high in omega-3 fatty acids—*flaxseeds, chia seeds and walnuts*—given their potent anti-inflammatory properties and ability to reduce harmful cytokine production. *Fiber-rich foods* are equally crucial, not only as bulking agents but also as they support our gut microbiome's beneficial bacteria.

For many individuals, it may also be important to *avoid gluten (mainly wheat, rye, and barley) and lactose from dairy products.* These products may be responsible for digestive issues, itching, skin rash, anxiety, or chronic fatigue. By avoiding these products, within few weeks you can notice significant improvement in your symptoms.

Gut Microbiome

The gut microbiome—which we'll explore more deeply later in this chapter—deserves special attention. This community of trillions of microorganisms serves as a key regulator of our immune system. Through years of treating patients, I've seen how a balanced microbiome helps manage immune responses effectively. I often recommend incorporating *probiotics* through fermented foods like yogurt, kefir, and sauerkraut, along with *prebiotics* that nourish beneficial bacteria. This approach consistently leads to a more balanced immune system and reduced chronic inflammation.

Exercise and Mindfulness

Strength exercises remain another cornerstone in reducing inflammation and enhancing longevity. The research confirms what I've observed clinically: regular physical activity lowers inflammatory markers and improves insulin sensitivity. Equally important is *stress management*—persistent stress elevates cortisol levels, directly fueling inflammation and compromising immune function. I've found that practices like mindfulness meditation, deep breathing, and adequate sleep are essential for maintaining balanced cortisol levels and reducing inflammation over time.

Medications

Regarding medications, several have proven effective in addressing systemic chronic inflammation—a condition I frequently see linked to age-related diseases like cardiovascular disease, diabetes, and neurodegenerative disorders. These medications, while not suitable for everyone, target inflammation at its root. Some are being investigated for their potential anti-aging benefits due to their role in reducing cellular damage from chronic inflammation.

Metformin particularly interests me as one of the most promising interventions. While primarily known as a diabetes medication, its benefits extend far beyond improving insulin sensitivity and lowering blood sugar. I've observed significant anti-inflammatory effects, with reductions in markers like C-reactive protein (CRP) and interleukin-6 (IL-6). By addressing both insulin resistance and inflammation, metformin shows promise in slowing down inflammaging—the inflammation associated with aging.

Nonsteroidal anti-inflammatory drugs (NSAIDs), especially aspirin, deserve mention for their anti-inflammatory effects. Through COX-2 inhibition, aspirin reduces inflammatory compounds and offers cardioprotective benefits. However, I always caution my patients about long-term NSAID use due to potential gastrointestinal and kidney complications. Similarly, while *corticosteroids* such as prednisone effectively reduce inflammation, I reserve these for short-term use given their side effects, including bone loss and weight gain.

Statins, best known for lowering LDL cholesterol, also have anti-inflammatory properties. By reducing CRP and other inflammatory markers, statins not only lower cholesterol but also help prevent cardiovascular disease by reducing inflammation and halting the progression of atherosclerosis.

Let's explore *low-dose naltrexone (LDN)*, a remarkable medication that has gained significant attention in the field of regenerative medicine for its unique effects on inflammation and immune regulation. While originally developed for treating addiction at higher doses, low-dose naltrexone demonstrates fascinating immunomodulatory properties. This medication works through a unique mechanism: by briefly blocking opioid receptors, it triggers an upregulation of endorphins and enkephalins, leading to a profound modulation of immune function.

What makes LDN particularly intriguing is its ability to reduce pro-inflammatory cytokines and regulate T-regulatory cells while simultaneously enhancing endogenous opioid production. Clinical evidence shows this leads to a reduction in systemic inflammation without suppressing essential immune functions. Through careful daily dosing in the range of 1 mg–8 mg, LDN achieves these beneficial effects while maintaining an excellent safety profile, making it a valuable tool in my approach to managing chronic inflammatory conditions and supporting overall immune balance. At such low doses, it helps manage atherosclerosis, autoimmune diseases, chronic diseases of aging, and chronic pain.

Just as willow bark (which contains the main ingredient in aspirin) has been used since the fifth century BC as a pain reliever, *colchicine* is also one of the oldest remedies still in use today. It is derived from the bulblike corms of the *Colchicum autumnale* plant, also known as autumn crocus. Its history goes back to the Ebers Papyrus, thought to be one of the oldest medical texts, dating from 1500 BC Egypt. Colchicine, traditionally known for treating acute gout, has emerged as a powerful tool in our fight against chronic inflammation.

This ancient medication operates through sophisticated mechanisms to dampen inflammatory cascades, and what's particularly intriguing is colchicine's ability to reduce pro-inflammatory cytokines and suppress NLRP3 inflammasome activation—a key driver of chronic inflammation. Recent clinical evidence demonstrates its broader therapeutic potential, especially in reducing cardiovascular events and systemic inflammation markers. My clinical experiences using this for diseases and longevity show significant improvements clinically and by biomarker tests. *At a low dose of 0.5mg a day*, colchicine provides targeted anti-inflammatory effects without compromising essential immune functions, making it an elegant solution for managing chronic inflammatory states.

Biologics are newer anti-inflammatory drugs targeting specific inflammatory pathways that are used in some people with specific indications, especially autoimmune diseases like rheumatoid arthritis. These drugs block pro-inflammatory cytokines like TNF-alpha or IL-1, providing targeted treatment for chronic inflammation.

Supplements and Herbs

As a physician integrating traditional with modern medicine, I want to share with you several powerful herbs that I've found effective in reducing chronic inflammation and immune system hyperactivity.

Let me start with *turmeric*, particularly its active compound curcumin, which is widely used in Indian cooking. *Curcumin* has a powerful anti-inflammatory effect in my practice, where it effectively inhibits inflammatory molecules and helps manage conditions ranging from arthritis to heart disease. Similarly, *ginger*, with its active compounds called gingerols, has consistently demonstrated the ability to reduce pro-inflammatory chemicals and oxidative stress. I've seen particular benefits with digestive issues and joint problems.

Also *resveratrol*, found in red wine and grapes, *quercetin* from apples and onions, and *CoQ10*—an antioxidant crucial for cellular energy production. These compounds work at the molecular level, effectively reducing oxidative stress and inhibiting inflammatory pathways.

Boswellia, also known as Indian frankincense, has impressed me with its effectiveness in reducing inflammation, especially in patients with arthritis and inflammatory bowel disease (IBD). Its active compounds, Boswellic acids, work by blocking inflammation-promoting enzymes, leading to reduced swelling and pain. *Green tea*, rich in EGCG, is another powerful tool in our anti-inflammatory arsenal. It has ability to lower inflammatory markers like C-reactive protein (CRP) while providing protection against oxidative damage.

I've found *holy basil (tulsi), called holy because it's sacred in Hinduism*, particularly valuable for managing both inflammation and stress. *Rosemary*, containing carnosol and rosmarinic acid, has shown promising results in reducing inflammation and supporting brain health. *Ashwagandha* has proven especially effective in balancing the immune system and cortisol levels, addressing inflammation linked to chronic stress. *Cloves*, with their active compound eugenol, have demonstrated particular efficacy in reducing joint inflammation while providing antioxidant protection.

I have seen that incorporating these herbs strategically into a patient's routine can effectively manage inflammation, and thus enhance youthful vitality, and promote longevity. I grew up using, and still do, many of these herbs in Indian cooking and as part of everyday living. *I particularly enjoy making fresh herbal tea myself, especially for my customary afternoon tea.* I keep it simple by boiling the water with some tulsi leaves, ginger, turmeric, clove, and cinnamon sticks—and optionally topping the brew with honey and lemon. At times I will add Darjeeling tea leaves in the mix. I find this fresh herbal tea both healing and refreshing. You should try it sometime and feel the serenity.

As we discussed above, through an *integrated approach* to managing chronic inflammation—combining advanced therapies with optimized lifestyle interventions—I've seen significant improvements in my patients' disease trajectories and healthspan. By addressing the root causes of chronic inflammation, we can slow down the aging process and improve the quality of life as we age.

Gut Health, Dysbiosis, Microbiome, and Leaky Gut

Science is proving what traditional East Indian medicine, Ayurveda, has known for millennia: your gut has deep influence on your immune cell function, metabolism, and even brain chemical modulation. Your gut is therefore called your "second brain," although a few of my Ayurvedic physician friends insist that it should be called the "first brain" instead. In recent years, gut health has emerged as one of the most critical factors influencing overall health, diseases, longevity, and youthfulness.

Now, I want to explore with you the critical role the gut plays in overall health, particularly in body's immune response and its connection to chronic inflammation. At the heart of gut health lies the *microbiome*, a vast ecosystem of trillions of bacteria, fungi, and microorganisms living symbiotically in the digestive tract. When in balance, the microbiome supports optimal health by promoting nutrient absorption, regulating immune responses, and producing essential compounds that reduce inflammation. However, when disrupted, this balance can lead to *dysbiosis*—an imbalance in gut bacteria that can trigger systemic health issues, including *leaky gut syndrome, chronic inflammation, and accelerated aging.*

> Research is clear that gut microbiome impacts health, disease, and aging by influencing immune cells, insulin resistance, mitochondrial function, inflammation, metabolism, and brain neurotransmitters.

It is helpful to clarify here an important distinction between two terms I discuss with patients: while *leaky gut* specifically refers to disruption in the intestinal lining causing increased permeability, *dysbiosis* describes an imbalance in gut bacteria composition. I've seen how dysbiosis often precedes and contributes to leaky gut, essentially making leaky gut a consequence of this bacterial imbalance. Given the importance of the gut's role in our health, let's talk about it in a little more detail.

- **Immunity and Disease Prevention:** The gut microbiome has a profound impact on immune function, with approximately 70 percent of immune cells residing in the gut. Beneficial bacteria influence immunity by promoting a tolerance to nonthreatening substances while enhancing our defense against pathogens through the gut-associated lymphoid tissue (GALT). What particularly interests me is how an optimal bacterial balance prevents chronic inflammation through the production of *short-chain fatty*

acids (SCFAs), fostering stronger immunity and lowering autoimmune disease risk.
- **Brain Health and Mental Well-Being:** The research on what is called "gut-brain axis" has revolutionized my approach to treating mental health conditions. This bidirectional communication system, linking the gastrointestinal system to the brain via the vagus nerve, plays a crucial role in health. Now here's where it gets more interesting still: the gut microbiome produces significant amounts of our neurotransmitters—serotonin, dopamine, and gamma-aminobutyric acid (GABA). In my clinical experience, I've observed how gut dysbiosis effects neuroinflammation and mental health disorders, potentially contributing to anxiety, depression, chronic stress, insomnia, and neurodegenerative diseases like Alzheimer's and Parkinson's.
- **Metabolic Health and Weight Regulation:** It is not commonly known that gut microbiota influences metabolic health, insulin resistance, and weight regulation. Certain gut bacteria assist in breaking down complex carbohydrates into *SCFAs*. These are fatty acids with two to six carbon atoms that are produced by bacterial fermentation by the gut microbiome and support insulin sensitivity and energy metabolism. An imbalanced gut leads to insulin resistance and obesity, while affecting appetite-regulating hormones like ghrelin and leptin.
- **Heart and Cardiovascular Health:** In my practice, I've seen how gut health significantly impacts cardiovascular function through its influence on cholesterol metabolism, blood pressure regulation, and systemic inflammation levels. SCFAs also lower cholesterol levels and reduce inflammation contributing to atherosclerosis, making gut health crucial for cardiovascular disease.
- **Longevity and Healthy Aging:** In focusing on longevity medicine, I've observed how gut health connects

to healthy aging through reducing chronic inflammation and supporting mitochondrial function. What fascinates me most is how a balanced microbiome reduces cellular senescence biomarkers, effectively delaying age-related cellular dysfunction while supporting stem cell activity crucial for tissue repair and regeneration.

- **Aging Skin:** The fine lines, dryness, and wrinkles that occur with aging are caused by multiple intrinsic and extrinsic factors. Both gut and skin microbiomes have protective roles, and an imbalance leads to an accelerated skin aging process. Interestingly, cosmetic companies are now developing products to improve the gut microbiome to enhance the skin's appearance.

Strategies to Help Gut Health and the Gut Microbiome

I've clinically seen how gut health profoundly impacts immunity, metabolism, brain health, and aging. I consistently advise following a gut-friendly lifestyle rich in fiber, prebiotics, and probiotics, while avoiding excessive antibiotics and processed foods. Science is clear—nurturing the gut microbiome is key to optimizing health and extending both healthspan and lifespan.

In the VitalLife program, restoring gut health and microbiome is a cornerstone for achieving optimal health, curing disease, and promoting longevity. By repairing the gut lining and rebalancing the microbiome, we can reverse the damaging effects of dysbiosis and leaky gut. It is good to start with certain specific microbiome tests, such as Viome and Ombre, widely used these days and few select inflammation markers.

Everything good and bad that you eat all day long is what really impacts your gut microbiome. Your diet plays a vital role in restoring and maintaining gut health, particularly in supporting a balanced microbiome and reducing chronic inflammation. The foods we consume directly influence the composition and diversity of the gut microbiome, which in turn affects digestion, immune function, and overall well-being. A *whole-food, plant-based diet* forms the foundation for a healthy gut, as it is rich in fiber, antioxidants, and prebiotics, all of which nourish beneficial gut bacteria and promote microbial diversity.

Fiber is not just a bulking agent; it is essential for gut health because it acts as fuel for the beneficial bacteria that reside in the colon. These bacteria ferment fiber, producing short-chain fatty acids (SCFAs) like butyrate, which have anti-inflammatory effects and help maintain the integrity of the gut lining. Foods high in fiber, such as leafy greens, legumes, whole grains, and nuts, support a diverse microbiome and prevent the overgrowth of harmful bacteria. Additionally, fiber helps regulate digestion and prevents constipation, which can otherwise disrupt the balance of gut bacteria.

Prebiotic foods are specific types of fiber that feed the good bacteria in the gut, promoting their growth and activity. Prebiotics, found in foods such as garlic, onions, leeks, asparagus, and bananas, *act as food for beneficial microbes, helping them thrive and outcompete harmful bacteria.* These foods also enhance the production of SCFAs, which further support the gut lining and reduce inflammation. By regularly consuming prebiotic-rich foods, individuals can encourage the growth of healthy bacterial strains like *Lactobacillus* and *Bifidobacterium*, which are critical for maintaining a healthy gut.

Probiotic-rich foods, such as yogurt, kefir, sauerkraut, kimchi, and other fermented vegetables introduce live beneficial bacteria into the digestive system. These probiotics help restore microbial diversity, especially after periods of stress, illness, or antibiotic use, which can deplete the microbiome. Probiotics not only help crowd out harmful bacteria but also support immune function by reinforcing the gut barrier and preventing the entry of harmful pathogens into the bloodstream.

In addition to fiber, prebiotics, and probiotics, *a diet rich in antioxidants* plays a vital role in gut health. Antioxidants from fruits and vegetables like berries, broccoli, spinach, and beets help neutralize harmful free radicals that can damage the gut lining and contribute to inflammation. Polyphenols, found in foods like green tea, dark chocolate, and grapes, also have anti-inflammatory properties and support a healthy microbiome by promoting the growth of beneficial bacteria. These compounds help protect the gut from oxidative stress, which can otherwise lead to leaky gut syndrome and systemic inflammation.

Moreover, the elimination of processed foods, unhealthy fats, and added sugars is equally important in supporting gut health. Highly processed foods and sugars can feed harmful bacteria, leading to dysbiosis and inflammation. Reducing the intake of these inflammatory foods while focusing on whole, unprocessed options allows the microbiome to thrive, creating a more balanced and resilient digestive system.

In addition to diet, certain *supplements* help repair the gut and support microbiome health. *L-glutamine* strengthens the intestinal lining, helping the body regenerate gut cells, while *zinc carnosine* and *collagen* promote healing of the gut barrier and reduce inflammation. *Probiotic supplements* with a broad spectrum of bacterial strains can restore balance in the gut, especially after periods of stress or illness, which often disrupt the microbiome.

Herbal medicine has long played a central role in gut health, particularly in traditional Indian Ayurvedic practices, which offer powerful remedies proven to support digestion, reduce inflammation, and restore balance to the gut microbiome. Several herbs stand out for their gut-friendly properties to help heal the gut and promote overall health.

As with so many other herbs and spices that I was introduced to when growing up in India, *triphala* (from Sanskrit language meaning *tri* for three, *phala* for fruits) has been an essential blend of herbs for my own gut health. If tolerated by patients,

I use triphala extensively. It is a traditional Ayurvedic blend of three fruits—*amalaki, bibhitaki,* and *haritaki*—and is renowned for its ability to support digestion, cleanse the intestines, and promote the growth of healthy, beneficial bacteria in the gut. Triphala acts as a gentle laxative, helping to remove toxins from the digestive tract while nourishing the gut lining. Its anti-inflammatory and antioxidant properties also support overall gut health by reducing oxidative stress and maintaining the integrity of the gut barrier.

Holy basil (tulsi) reduces cortisol and soothes inflammation, protecting the gut from stress-related damage. It calms digestion and supports the gut-brain axis, enhancing gut health. *Ashwagandha* lowers cortisol, preventing stress-induced dysbiosis, while its anti-inflammatory effects protect the gut lining and reduce leaky gut symptoms. *Turmeric* and its active compound, *curcumin*, reduce inflammation in the gut and help repair damage, strengthening the gut lining and improving microbiome balance. *Cumin* stimulates digestive enzymes and reduces bloating, improving nutrient absorption and protecting the gut from harmful bacteria. *Asafetida* is a natural remedy for bloating and digestive discomfort, with antimicrobial properties that support a healthy microbiome. *Saffron* offers anti-inflammatory benefits, protecting the gut lining and supporting mood regulation through the gut-brain axis.

In addition to these herbs, addressing dysbiosis and leaky gut involves *minimizing exposure to gut disruptors like chronic stress, antibiotics, and environmental toxins.* Chronic stress has a direct impact on gut health, weakening the intestinal barrier and promoting dysbiosis. Stress reduction techniques, including yoga, meditation, and deep breathing, have been shown to support gut health by lowering cortisol levels and enhancing gut-brain communication.

These strategies offer a holistic approach to restoring gut health and improving overall well-being. In some advanced cases, innovative treatments like *fecal microbiota transplantation (FMT)* may be used to repopulate the gut with healthy bacteria, especially in individuals with severe dysbiosis. Though this therapy is still emerging, its potential for restoring the microbiome and improving gut health is promising.

The connection between gut health and overall vitality is undeniable. Through the strategies incorporated into the VitalLife program, so many individuals have experienced significant improvements in energy levels, cognitive clarity, and overall well-being. By addressing dysbiosis, leaky gut, and maintaining a balanced microbiome, you can protect against inflammation, promote youthfulness, and support a longer, healthier life.

—

As we close this chapter on the holistic approach to immune health and gut vitality, it becomes clear that nurturing these systems is crucial for achieving longevity and reversing diseases. These integrative strategies—rooted in both ancient wisdom and modern science—empower your body to thrive, extending your healthspan and ensuring that the journey of aging is met with vitality, not decline.

As we move forward, we enter the world of personalized compounded pharmacy medicines, tailored to your unique biology and needs. In the next chapter, we'll explore how these custom formulations can transform your health in ways that go far beyond conventional medicine.

CHAPTER 14

Ultra-Personalized Compounded Medications

In life, pain is inevitable, suffering is optional.
—*Buddhist proverb*

The art of medicine consists of amusing the patient while nature cures the disease.
—*Voltaire, French writer (1694–1778)*

Over the years, I've observed a significant shift from standardized medical protocols to precision medicine, which leverages individual biological markers to optimize therapeutic outcomes. This approach aligns with my consistent belief that each patient's unique biochemical and cellular profile requires personalized intervention strategies. Pharmaceutical compounding, performed by specialized FDA-approved US facilities, stands at the forefront of this personalization revolution, creating precisely calibrated formulations tailored to individual patient needs.

When evaluating patients for personalized pharmacy protocols for longevity, *first I meticulously analyze their biomarkers, including those for hormonal cascades, metabolic efficiency, and cellular regeneration capacity*. This comprehensive assessment often reveals subtle biochemical variations that demand precise therapeutic adjustments, which are impossible to achieve with standard pharmaceutical dosing. Compounded medications *allow for exact calibration* of bioactive compounds, optimizing hormone levels, incorporating specific peptide sequences, and engineering novel drug delivery systems.

I have witnessed how customized care surpasses traditional pharmacies, which provide only mass-produced medications in fixed dosages. Pharmaceutical compounding offers a level of control and precision that has revolutionized my practice, allowing patients to experience faster results, fewer side effects, and a more sustainable path to health.

As I have been utilizing in VitalLife, compounding pharmacies *also enable innovation in delivery methods*, from transdermal creams and sublingual tablets to injectable formulations and time-released capsules. These options can improve patient adherence and overall outcomes, particularly in anti-aging medicine, where consistency and precision are crucial for long-term success. The rise of personalized medicine, powered by certified compounding pharmacies, represents a new frontier in healthcare that extends lifespan and improves healthspan.

In addition to the various hormones and peptides we explored in chapter 11, such as testosterone, estrogen blockers, and bioidentical hormones for women, there's an exciting array of other compounds that can be tailored specifically to your needs. What's even more convenient is that *many of these treatments can be combined into single formulations*, making them easier to use and manage as part of a comprehensive health regimen. These custom treatments extend beyond the basics of hormone replacement, offering targeted solutions for longevity, vitality, sexual health, and even immune system support. With all these personalized options, you can take charge of your health in a way that truly meets your unique needs and goals.

I have found that integrating these custom formulations with comprehensive lifestyle modifications—including targeted nutritional interventions, structured exercise protocols, and sleep hygiene optimization—creates synergistic effects that enhance therapeutic outcomes. This integrated approach consistently yields sustainable improvements in both objective biomarkers and subjective measures of vitality and health optimization.

I have deliberately omitted the dosing schedule for many of these products I discuss below, because all treatments need to be customized by an experienced physician based on an individual person's clinical history, biomarker and other tests, personal goals, and medical needs.

Rapamycin: A Senolytic Compound

As a physician dedicated to longevity medicine, I find the discovery story of rapamycin quite fascinating. It begins in one of Earth's most isolated locations—Easter Island—where researchers in the 1960s isolated a remarkable bacterium, *Streptomyces hygroscopicus*, from the soil. The compound they derived, named rapamycin after the island's native name, Rapa Nui, initially appeared promising as an antifungal agent. The therapeutic potential of rapamycin expanded dramatically, first proving invaluable as an immunosuppressant for preventing organ rejection in transplant patients through its potent T cell modulation.

What truly excites me about rapamycin is its profound impact on cellular aging through selective inhibition of a protein complex, mTORC1, within the mTOR (mechanistic target of rapamycin) pathway. This pathway orchestrates cellular nutrient sensing, protein synthesis, and *autophagy* (cellular processes that break down and recycle parts of old cells)—fundamental processes in metabolism and aging. When this mTOR pathway is overactive, it suppresses autophagy and promotes cellular senescence, which contributes to accelerated aging and age-related pathologies.

When we examine its senolytic benefits, recent research shows that rapamycin effectively reduces senescent cells and the associated chronic inflammation, a primary driver of aging and age-related diseases. Through careful clinical application, we can harness rapamycin's ability to modulate overactive mTOR signaling, so that it encourages damaged cells to either repair themselves through enhanced autophagy or undergo *apoptosis* (programmed cell death), creating an environment where healthier cells can thrive. This cellular optimization helps improve tissue function and delay onset of conditions like diabetes, cognitive decline, and cardiovascular issues.

The research data supporting rapamycin's potential is evolving, especially in animal research. Studies from the National Institute on Aging demonstrated a 10–30 percent *lifespan extension in mice* when administered later in life. What I find even more relevant to my clinical practice is the improvement in healthspan markers—these mice didn't just live longer, they maintained better mitochondrial function, glucose homeostasis, and reduced incidence of age-related diseases, including heart issues, cancer, and neurodegeneration. This is only animal data, however, and requires us to be careful in translating to human use. *Human use data is limited*, yet experience by clinicians from around the world so far has been quite encouraging, especially considering the lack of serious side effects when used in low, once weekly doses.

Through careful compounding, we can create tailored formulations that allow for *intermittent microdosing* (for example, 4–8 mg once a week, with eight weeks on and eight weeks off, as a *cyclical regimen*. This is often the *optimal approach for harnessing anti-aging benefits while minimizing immunosuppressive effects*. In my practice, I've seen improvements in key biomarkers: optimized metabolic parameters and reduced inflammatory markers. These benefits may extend to improved mitochondrial function, insulin resistance, and potentially even lifespan extension, especially when used as a part of comprehensive protocol. However, I always emphasize that while rapamycin offers these exciting benefits, *proper medical oversight with regular monitoring of biomarkers remains essential for optimal outcomes*.

Side effects to watch for include mouth sores, increased risk of infection, or disruptions in lipid levels. Because rapamycin can suppress immune function, it's crucial to use it under medical supervision to ensure you're getting the benefits without compromising your health. The best way to use rapamycin is to start with a low dose and gradually adjust based on your response, needs, and side effects, if any. I suggest using it in cycles rather than continuously, allowing your body time to adapt and recover.

Compounded Oral Ketamine for Microdosing Protocol

In my clinical practice, while exploring the latest therapeutics for neuropsychiatric disorders, I've observed profound transformations through psychedelic medicine, particularly ketamine. Building on our earlier discussions of psychedelic compounds in chapter 10, I've seen these substances demonstrate remarkable efficacy across a spectrum of conditions—from treatment-resistant depression and anxiety to complex neurological disorders. What fascinates me most is their potential role in longevity medicine through their unique ability to promote both psychological and physiological healing mechanisms.

The therapeutic application of ketamine through precision microdosing, particularly in compounded formulations, represents a significant advancement in treating conditions I frequently encounter: for instance, *treatment-resistant depression, anxiety disorders, PTSD, and chronic pain syndromes*. It has been reported in scientific literature that subtherapeutic doses of ketamine significantly enhance *neuroplasticity*—promoting dendritic spine growth and synaptic remodeling—leading to profound improvements in cognitive and emotional processing.

The precision of compounded ketamine for microdosing protocols is crucial for optimal outcomes. Through careful formulation, we can create patient-specific dosing regimens that maintain cognitive clarity while promoting emotional healing, without inducing dissociative effects. I've successfully utilized various administration routes in my practice—including *sublingual tablets, intranasal delivery systems, and oral troches*—each offering distinct pharmacokinetic advantages for at-home administration.

The clinical results continue to impress me: patients consistently report enhanced mood stability, reduced anxiety levels, and improved emotional regulation. What's particularly noteworthy is the consistent feedback about increased present-moment awareness, enhanced emotional openness, and deeper interpersonal connections—therapeutic effects that I've observed contribute significantly to sustained emotional resilience and healing.

As we discussed in chapter 10, in my practice, I've seen results using two distinct approaches. The first is *intermittent dosing protocols*, where we use therapeutic doses to actively manage various conditions by giving a dose three times a week. It's often administered in cycles, with a few weeks on followed by breaks to allow the body and mind to integrate the benefits. This approach helps to maximize ketamine's therapeutic effects while minimizing the risks.

The second approach, which particularly excites me, is daily *microdosing or very-low-dose (VLD) therapy*. This gentler method works wonderfully for treatment of many conditions, including phobias, social anxiety, eating disorders, obsessive-compulsive disorder, and anxiety. It has also shown intriguing potential for anti-aging benefits.

> Microdosing with oral ketamine might provide anti-aging benefits, especially when combined with other products such as rapamycin, metformin, LDN, sermorelin, NAD+, and supplements, among others.

Of course, as with any treatment, there are *side effects* to watch out for. While the microdoses are generally well tolerated, some people may experience mild dizziness, nausea, or a feeling of dissociation. Because ketamine can affect your mental state, it's crucial that it's used under the guidance of a healthcare provider. Another thing to watch for is the potential for dependency, though this is typically more of a concern with higher doses. Regular check-ins with your doctor are important to monitor your progress and make any necessary adjustments.

I highly recommend combining ketamine microdosing with psychotherapy, meditation, or mindfulness practices, which can deepen the healing process and create long-lasting improvements in mental and emotional health. And, as in VitalLife, always use it as a part of comprehensive strategic plan.

Low-Dose Naltrexone: A Potent Anti-inflammation Medicine

Low-dose naltrexone (LDN) is an exciting, relatively unconventional therapy that's gaining a lot of attention in the world of autoimmune and chronic illness treatment. Originally developed as a medication to block the effects of opioids, naltrexone at full doses has been used for decades to treat addiction. However, in low doses, as I use in my practice, it does something entirely different—it works by calming an overactive immune system, reducing inflammation, and promoting the body's natural ability to heal itself.

With a low dose, it boosts endorphin production, which not only regulates immune function but also enhances mood, alleviates pain, and improves overall energy levels. This makes it particularly effective for individuals managing autoimmune conditions like rheumatoid arthritis, multiple sclerosis, Crohn's disease, and even post-viral syndromes such as long COVID. It's also beneficial for those suffering from fibromyalgia and chronic fatigue syndrome.

In my clinical experience, results from LDN are enhanced when used with other inflammatory strategies as discussed in the previous chapter, including compounds such as colchicine and metformin.

In its compounded form, I can easily customize low-dose naltrexone for each individual, allowing for the exact dose a person needs to support healing without the side effects that come with higher doses. LDN is usually taken *orally*, either as tablets, capsules or in liquid form, typically at night. In my practice, I've witnessed remarkable transformations—many patients report significant improvements in their symptoms within just a few months, particularly *in managing chronic pain and inflammation as in auto-immune diseases and many chronic illnesses, including cardiovascular disease.*

As with any medication, there are *side effects* to watch for, though LDN is generally very well tolerated. Some people may experience sleep disturbances or vivid dreams when they first start taking it, but these usually subside as the body adjusts. Occasionally, mild headaches or digestive upset can occur, but serious side effects are rare. It's important to monitor how your body responds and adjust the dose if needed, always under the guidance of an experienced healthcare provider.

The best way to use LDN is to *start with a low dose (0.5 to 1.5 mg a day) and gradually increase it to 6 to 8 mg a day*, allowing the body to adjust and maximize its immune-modulating benefits. *It works best when combined with other treatments that support overall health*, like anti-inflammatory diets, supplements, and stress-reduction techniques. The key with LDN is patience—since it works by slowly rebalancing the immune system, it may take a few months to see its full effects. But I can tell you from my experience that for many people, the results are worth the wait.

Sermorelin: A Natural Growth Hormone Booster Peptide

Clinical experience with peptide therapeutics shows sermorelin represents a fascinating advancement in our approach to endocrine optimization. As a synthetic peptide analog, it demonstrates remarkable efficacy in age-management protocols. The compelling aspect of sermorelin lies in its physiological mechanism—rather than introducing an exogenous growth hormone, *it stimulates the pituitary gland to enhance endogenous growth hormone production.* I appreciate this biomimetic approach because it offers superior safety profiles by preserving the body's natural feedback mechanisms, rather than disrupting endocrine pathways with synthetic growth hormone injections.

Through careful titration, we can optimize dosing based on individual patient requirements. *Subcutaneous administration, or oral formulations*, which I prefer, are typically recommended. These are strategically timed for evening administration to align with natural circadian growth hormone secretion. When used as part of a comprehensive hormone and peptide optimization protocol, the *therapeutic benefits* I see in clinical practice include enhanced muscle mass and strength that helps counter sarcopenia, boosted overall energy level, decreased fat percentage, better mental focus, enhanced metabolism, improved sleep patterns, accelerated recovery, improved skin elasticity, and even increased bone mineralization.

When evaluating sermorelin therapy, understanding *potential adverse effects* remains crucial. While clinical experience shows excellent tolerability profiles, careful monitoring for common reactions like injection site inflammation, cephalgia, or transient vertigo is essential. In a smaller subset of patients, mild peripheral edema or arthralgia symptoms may occur, though these typically respond well to dosage modifications. Implementing rigorous monitoring protocols ensures therapeutic efficacy while minimizing adverse effects.

Treatment protocols typically span several months, recognizing that the gradual enhancement of endogenous growth hormone production, while slower than direct hormone supplementation, offers superior physiological benefits and safety profiles.

Intravenous (IV) Infusion Therapies

Compounded IV infusion therapies have become a quite popular and effective way *to deliver a powerful blend of vitamins, minerals, and cellular nutrients directly into the bloodstream.* I have now seen so many different retail centers, spas, physician offices, resorts, and even home-based outfits providing IV therapies. I recently heard of an entrepreneur in Las Vegas who decided to capitalize on providing these IV therapies to tourists in hotel rooms around town in order to treat hangovers after drinking and partying. Pretty targeted approach to monetize, I imagine.

The pharmacokinetic advantages of parenteral delivery ensure superior bioavailability through direct systemic administration, circumventing enterohepatic circulation and ensuring immediate cellular availability. In clinical practice, this direct-to-circulation pathway demonstrates markedly enhanced therapeutic efficiency compared with traditional oral supplementation routes.

I think the best part is that the precision of compounded IV formulations allows for a sophisticated therapeutic customization based on your specific biochemical requirements and clinical objectives. Protocol designs typically incorporate key therapeutic agents: *high-dose ascorbic acid* for immune modulation, *B-complex vitamins* for cellular energetics and neurotransmitter optimization, *glutathione* for cellular detoxification and matrix integrity, NAD+ for athletic performance and recovery, and targeted amino acid profiles supporting muscle repair and tissue regeneration. *Anti-aging protocol* focusses on specific nutrient combination of vitamins, minerals and amino acids to enhance cellular renewal, mitigate oxidative stress cascades, and optimize collagen synthesis pathways.

The therapeutic benefits of IV infusion protocols are extensive. *For immunity*, these infusions can help reduce the severity and duration of illnesses, strengthen the body's natural defenses, and support faster recovery from infections. *For anti-aging*, they provide antioxidants that fight free radicals, slow down the aging process, and support healthier skin and hair. I also find IV infusion beneficial when athletes or those with active lifestyles use these therapies *to speed up recovery* after physical exertion, repair muscle tissue, and reduce inflammation. Additionally, many people experience *increased energy levels, improved mental clarity, and better hydration*, making them feel more vibrant and rejuvenated. These outcomes reflect the sophisticated interplay between precise nutrient delivery and cellular optimization, establishing IV therapy as a cornerstone in advanced preventive medicine protocols.

As with any therapy, there are best practices to follow for IV infusions. It's important to work with an experienced healthcare provider who can assess your needs and customize the right blend of nutrients for you. Since each infusion is tailored to the individual, regular monitoring and adjustments may be necessary to ensure you're getting the most benefit from your treatments. *Most people receive IV infusions on a weekly or biweekly basis*, depending on their health goals and how their body responds.

Staying hydrated, eating a nutrient-rich diet, using targeted supplements and maintaining a balanced lifestyle will further enhance the benefits of these infusions, allowing your body to make the most of the nutrients it receives. When done properly as part of a comprehensive treatment plan, compounded IV infusions can be a game-changer in optimizing health, longevity, and overall well-being.

NAD+: A New Fountain of Youth?

I have found NAD+ to be an interesting compounded product with broad clinical applications, and I incorporate this for many patients starting on VitalLife. NAD stands for nicotinamide adenine dinucleotide, and the plus sign indicates an oxidized form when NAD loses an electron. NADH is a reduced form of the molecule, which means that it gains the electron lost by NAD+. It is an essential coenzyme that drives key cellular processes and plays a critical role in converting food into energy. Higher levels of NAD+ can increase overall quality of life by *improving mitochondrial function and energy production.*

It also aids in repairing DNA damage and promoting healthy cell function, which is necessary for overall health and healthy aging. A decline in NAD+ levels has been linked to age-related diseases, but researchers have found NAD+ therapy to potentially slow down the aging process.

NAD+ therapy has remarkable breadth of potential therapeutic benefits, including athletic performance, cognitive improvement; reversal of aging signs; prevention of age-induced diseases such as heart disease, diabetes, and cancer; and possibly increasing lifespan. It helps maintain youthful skin and hair texture, and boosts cell energy production. It also *activates sirtuins*, which regulate cell metabolism, prevent chronic inflammation, and boost immunity.

NAD+ precursors are substances that can be converted into NAD+ in the body, and they play a crucial role in maintaining healthy levels of the coenzyme. Common NAD+ precursors include niacin, nicotinamide riboside (NR), tryptophan, pyridoxal 5′-phosphate (PLP), and nicotinamide mononucleotide (NMN). *Niacin* is found in foods like tuna and avocados, while NR occurs naturally in milk and yeast and is available as a supplement. *Tryptophan* is an amino acid found in proteins, and *PLP*, which is the active form of vitamin B_6, is found in nuts, seeds, and whole grains. The effectiveness of tryptophan as a supplement requires further research, and PLP must be activated with magnesium before it can convert into NAD+. *NMN* is a primary precursor for NAD+ and has been found effective against oxidative stress and DNA damage in small clinical trials and animal studies.

Although NAD+ precursors are available in small amounts in various foods, taking supplements may be necessary to increase NAD+ levels. While these precursors offer numerous benefits, caution is advised when taking NR supplements with blood pressure medication.

NAD+ therapy can be administered orally, through nasal spray, transdermally, subcutaneously, or intravenously as an injection or IV drip. Oral administration is safer, more affordable, and more comfortable for self-administration, but it is metabolized quickly, so its effect lasts only for a short time. I recommend nasal spray for individuals with severe health issues as it is easy to self-administer but still allows quicker access to brain cells. Transdermal cream can also be applied to your skin for anti-aging effects especially around the face and via patches to be absorbed systematically.

I prefer subcutaneous and IV methods that I believe provide better and faster results, but they are more expensive and can have adverse side effects such as abdominal pain, brain fog, bruising, cramping, diarrhea, fatigue, headaches, nausea, and redness or swelling at the injection site. While mostly safe when administered by medical professionals, you should be aware of the side effects.

Lots of medspas and clinics offer this as IV therapy. Like so many other treatments, *NAD+ treatments are not right for everyone and should not be used as a solitary treatment modality.* When considering NAD+ therapy, it is crucial that you first consult with a healthcare professional, who can advise whether or not NAD+ therapy is the right course of action for your particular needs and health condition. It is important to find a reputable provider in your area specializing in this treatment. It is also helpful to look into what other people have experienced when using NAD+ therapy and if any reviews are available.

Glutathione: The "Master Antioxidant"

Glutathione is a powerful compound made from amino acids glycine, cysteine and glutamic acid. It plays a critical role in *detoxification, immune function, and cellular repair.* It's naturally produced in the body and works by neutralizing free radicals, supporting the body's defense against oxidative stress, and promoting the healthy functioning of cells. Over time, however, our natural levels of glutathione can be depleted due to aging, stress, illness, processed foods, alcohol use, or smoking. This is where compounded glutathione come into play—it offers a way to replenish glutathione levels and boost the body's ability to detoxify and repair itself from within.

In the form of a compounded injection, glutathione is delivered directly into the bloodstream, allowing for maximum absorption and effectiveness. This method bypasses the digestive system, which can limit the amount of glutathione that actually reaches your cells when taken orally. Injections are commonly used for their *detoxification benefits*, helping the liver eliminate toxins more effectively, as well as for *skin health* (some people report a brighter, more even complexion) and to *improve energy levels*. Glutathione is also a powerful *supporter of immune function*, helping the body fight off infections and recover more quickly from illness. I find that athletes or individuals under high stress see marked improvements in recovery and reduced inflammation.

While generally considered safe, there are a few *side effects* to keep in mind. Some people may experience mild injection site irritation or allergic reactions, though these are rare. Other potential side effects could include bloating or cramps, but these are typically mild and short-lived. Because glutathione is such a powerful antioxidant, it's important to use glutathione infusion under the guidance of an experienced healthcare provider to ensure that the dose is right for you, and to monitor its effects over time.

For best results, I recommend glutathione injections through a series of intravenous infusion sessions, often spaced out over several weeks. Depending on your health goals—whether it's detoxification, immune support, or anti-aging—you and your doctor can determine the right frequency and dosage. For many, *it works best when combined with other therapies*, like IV infusions of NAD+, vitamins or other antioxidants, to provide comprehensive support for overall health and vitality. Incorporating a healthy lifestyle, rich in fruits and vegetables, will also help to support your body's natural production of glutathione and extend the benefits of these injections over the long term.

Compounded Hormones and Peptides

We discussed this important element of the VitalLife program in detail in chapter 11—hormone and peptide optimization is a step beyond conventional hormone replacement therapy. The customization used in the program is influenced by several factors, including lab data, the severity of symptoms, the chosen route of administration (oral, cream, pellets, or injections), and any underlying medical conditions. We have also discussed how *equally important it is to incorporate support for the metabolic system, gut health, and cellular mitochondrial function.* These are foundational elements that determine how efficiently your body utilizes the hormones and peptides introduced during therapy.

It is important to always consult with an expert healthcare provider to ensure that these treatments are right for you and to receive the correct dosage and guidance for safe, effective use. Below are some of the key compounded products I use in my practice to address hormone and peptide optimization for both men and women:

Hormones and Peptides for Men

Testosterone: The four primary forms of testosterone hormone used are testosterone enanthate, testosterone cypionate, testosterone propionate, and testosterone undecanoate. In addition to injections, testosterone can also be delivered through various alternative methods, such as oral tablets, buccal tablets, transdermal gels, patches, solutions, and pellets implanted under the skin for a long-lasting, steady release of the hormone. I usually select the specific method of administration based on individual preferences, convenience, lifestyle, and overall health considerations.

Estrogen Blockers: There are two primary types of estrogen blockers used in men's hormone therapy: aromatase inhibitors, such as anastrozole (Arimidex), letrozole, and exemestane; and selective estrogen receptor modulators (SERMs), such as tamoxifen and clomiphene (Clomid).

HCG: It is used in testosterone optimization therapy to maintain testicular function, prevent atrophy, and preserve fertility by mimicking luteinizing hormone (LH). It stimulates natural testosterone production, complementing exogenous testosterone therapy.

Gonadorelin: It stimulates the pituitary gland to release LH and FSH, supporting natural testosterone and sperm production. It's ideal for men focused on preserving fertility or testicular health.

Oxytocin Nasal Spray: Oxytocin, also called the "bonding or love hormone"—because it increases intimacy, passion, and pleasure, and decreases stress and anxiety—is generally well tolerated and safe but should not be used more frequently than is prescribed, as a person can become dependent on the mood-elevating effect of this medication. It is most commonly used in spray or oral form.

Trimix: An injectable solution for men, highly effective for erectile dysfunction, it is a mix of three compounds (thus the name)—alprostadil, papaverine, and phentolamine.

PT-141: Popularly known as bremelanotide, this peptide improves libido. PT-141 is available in oral and injectable formulations, and can be combined with Cialis and oxytocin for optimal results.

Sermorelin: As discussed earlier, this peptide boosts your natural growth hormone levels. It is available in subcutaneous and oral form. Helps with lean muscle mass, energy metabolism, cellular regeneration, and sexual function.

Hormones and Peptides for Women

Bioidentical hormones are synthetic compounds that are derived from plant sources such as yams and soy and processed in labs to be identical to natural hormones produced by the human body. These include estrogen, testosterone, and progesterone. These hormones can be administered through various methods, including pills, patches, creams, or pellets, and are commonly used to treat symptoms of menopause, hormone imbalances, and other endocrine-related conditions. It's important to note that, like any hormone therapy, bioidentical hormones should be prescribed and monitored by an expert healthcare provider, as they can carry risks and potential side effects. For women struggling with vaginal symptoms, vaginal cream can be a good option.

Estrogen: Bioidentical estradiol, the most potent form of estrogen naturally found in women, is commonly prescribed in compounded formulations. Available forms include transdermal creams or gels, patches, vaginal tablets or creams, and oral capsules. Benefits include relief from hot flashes, night sweats, vaginal dryness, mood changes, and protection against bone loss. Dosing varies based on symptoms, age, and whether applied locally or systemically, with lower doses often used for vaginal symptoms alone. The transdermal route is often preferred as it bypasses liver metabolism and may carry lower risks than oral administration. To make it easier for patients to administer, *I can combine various doses of estradiol with progesterone and testosterone in one formulation.* Regular monitoring of symptoms and hormone levels is needed and helps optimize therapy while minimizing risks.

Progesterone: Bioidentical progesterone from compounding pharmacies is available in several formulations: oral capsules, vaginal suppositories, and transdermal creams. Benefits include improved sleep, reduced anxiety, menstrual regulation, decreased hot flashes, and vaginal health. For women on estrogen, it provides uterine protection. Unlike synthetic progestins, bioidentical progesterone typically carries fewer risks while effectively managing menopausal symptoms.

Testosterone: When prescribed for women, testosterone is delivered in much lower doses than for men, typically through creams, gels, or pellets, with careful monitoring to prevent masculinizing side effects. It affects not just libido but also muscle mass, bone density, cognitive function, and energy levels. Women's testosterone can decline with age, menopause, surgery, medications, or stress. Dosing must be precise to avoid side effects like acne or facial hair growth while still achieving benefits like improved mental clarity and energy. Regular blood monitoring is essential to maintain optimal hormone balance.

Oxytocin: Discussed above, the oral or spray form is also used for women to increase intimacy and pleasure.

PT-141: As discussed above, it's a peptide that is also used for women for similar benefits and may also be effective after menopause. It is available as oral and injectable formulation and can be combined with Cialis and oxytocin for optimal results. This combination can be quite effective for women with hypoactive sexual desire disorder (HSDD).

Sermorelin: As discussed above, sermorelin can also be prescribed for women for similar benefits.

In this chapter, we explored the powerful world of compounded medicine and how it can be tailored to meet the unique needs of each individual. From personalized hormone optimization protocols to advanced therapies like rapamycin, ketamine, low-dose naltrexone, sermorelin, and IV infusions, these novel solutions in VitalLife offer a comprehensive approach to improving health and vitality. *By working with FDA-certified, US-based compounding pharmacies,* we can fine-tune medications to support everything from immune function and cellular repair to health and anti-aging—ensuring that each patient's treatment is precisely matched to their goals.

As we move forward to the next section of this book, it's essential to understand that true health doesn't rely solely on medications or regenerative products. Lifestyle modifications—including a nutrient-rich diet, the right supplements, and a focus on exercise for strength and resilience—are just as crucial in maintaining optimal health, youthfulness, and longevity. The next part of this book will dive into these lifestyle pillars, exploring how they not only support physical health but also play a key role in enhancing emotional well-being and creating a foundation for a vibrant, fulfilling life at any age.

PART 4

LIFESTYLE CHANGES FOR ENDLESS YOUTHFULNESS

CHAPTER 15

Embracing a Plant-Based Diet: Improve Life and Longevity

When diet is wrong, medicine is of no use. When diet is correct, medicine is of no need.
—*Ayurvedic proverb*

He who takes medicine and neglects diet wastes the skills of his doctors.
—*Chinese proverb*

Ramesh, fifty-six, had immigrated from India at the age of twenty-two and fully embraced America, including the American diet. He was a successful businessman who owned several international brand hotels. He was living the American dream, or that's what he thought until eight years ago, when he was diagnosed with diabetes and high blood pressure. He was overweight and had high cholesterol. He had also developed peripheral neuropathy, which caused tingling in his legs. Despite constant supervision by his specialists and medical treatments, a few years later he developed chest pain and underwent a coronary angioplasty procedure with stent placement to reopen the blocked arteries in his heart.

A year before seeking my guidance, he underwent his third heart procedure—yet another attempt to clear blockages and implant stents in his coronary arteries. Despite the efforts of a team of specialists and a regimen of multiple medications, his health stubbornly defied improvement. His blood pressure and blood sugar levels remained alarmingly elevated, leaving him caught in a relentless cycle of fatigue, weakness, and despair.

At this point, every day was a struggle for him. Exhaustion consumed him, headaches pounded incessantly, and recurring chest pain served as a grim and constant reminder of his fragility. Anxiety became his constant companion—an unrelenting fear of next heart attack that might strike without warning and end his life. When his doctors told him there was nothing more they could do, he was left grappling with a devastating sense of helplessness and uncertainty, wondering if this was the life he was destined to endure.

When Ramesh walked into my clinic, he was at a pivotal crossroads in his life—a moment where he was ready to embrace any path that might restore his health and vitality. Following a comprehensive biomarker analysis that included biological age methylation test, I guided him toward a transformative plan: a strict whole-food, plant-based diet, entirely free of oil, processed foods, and anything fried. Paired with thirty minutes of daily exercise, carefully selected supplements, and an advanced anti-inflammatory protocol, the results that followed were nothing short of extraordinary.

In less than three months, Ramesh had shed twenty pounds and was able to eliminate several of his prescription medications for diabetes, blood pressure, and cholesterol. His energy surged back, empowering him to rediscover activities he had long abandoned. For the first time in years, he felt hopeful—confident that he was on a path of recovery, and optimistic about the future that lay ahead.

The transformation didn't just change Ramesh's life—it inspired those around him as well. During one of his follow-up visits to my clinic, his son revealed that he, too, had adopted the plant-based lifestyle after witnessing the profound changes in his father. Ramesh's journey became more than a personal victory—it sparked a ripple effect of inspiration and possibility within him.

With a whole-food, plant-based diet with no processed food, just like Ramesh, you too can decrease weight, improve blood sugar levels, control blood pressure better, and decrease cholesterol levels. I have seen many patients just like Ramesh who are able to decrease, and sometimes completely stop, their medications for diabetes, hypertension, cholesterol, and peripheral neuropathy after switching to a whole-food, plant-based diet with no processed food. In this chapter, we will explore the profound benefits of this approach and how it can be a key factor in your journey to longevity and improved healthspan.

Like so many of you, for me nutrition has always been the cornerstone of optimal health and wellness. Food is foundational to any optimal health and longevity protocol, and this is especially true for VitalLife. We all recognize the critical role of diet, supplements, and herbs in promoting vitality and extending lifespan. A healthy diet is one of the most powerful tools for enhancing energy, longevity, and overall well-being. What you eat doesn't just fuel your body—it directly shapes how well you age, how vibrant you feel, and how effectively your internal systems function.

I believe *what you eat (or drink) is THE most powerful medicine you prescribe yourself to enhance your healthspan and promote longevity*. Every bite you eat creates a biochemical reaction in your body that can either heal or harm, energize or exhaust, build or destroy every single cell in your body. Whatever you eat, ask yourself: *Are you eating for taste, pleasure, or because you're in a rush? Or are you eating to nourish your future self?*

Instead of the processed, calorie-dense diet that has regrettably become our staple these days, a *nutrient-dense diet*—rich in fresh fruits, fresh vegetables, whole grains, plant-based proteins, and healthy fats—provides the body with essential vitamins, minerals, and antioxidants that support optimal health. These foods work together to reduce inflammation, enhance immune function, and protect against chronic diseases such as heart disease, stroke, diabetes, and cancer.

It's not just about what you should eat, but even more importantly, understanding what you can't afford to eat. By focusing on whole, plant-based foods and minimizing exposure to processed foods and toxins such as pesticides, hormones, and preservatives in our food, we can support our body's natural healing processes and *enhance overall vitality, reverse diseases, and live longer.*

Diets: West Versus East

For the most part, there have been two predominant perspectives on health and nutrition across the world. The Western approach often relies on fast-acting pharmaceuticals and medical interventions to address health, disease, and wellness. In contrast, the Eastern world, including Mediterranean cultures, tends to respect nutrition as a primary driver of health and disease prevention.

The stark contrast between Western diets and Eastern (including Mediterranean) diets reveals much about their impact on health, disease, and longevity. The typical Western diet is characterized by *calorie-dense food* with high consumption of processed foods, refined sugars, processed fats, and processed meats. Fast food, sugary beverages, and ultra-processed snacks dominate this dietary landscape, leading to excessive calorie intake with minimal nutritional value. This results in deficiencies in essential nutrients like fiber, vitamins, and antioxidants, while contributing to chronic inflammation and insulin resistance, causing diseases. *The Western diet's reliance on convenience over quality has been linked to a rise in conditions such as obesity, heart disease, stroke, type 2 diabetes, and certain cancers.*

In contrast, Eastern and Mediterranean diets *emphasize nutrient-dense, whole, minimally processed foods* that nourish the body and support longevity. These diets are rich in fresh fruits, vegetables, whole grains, beans, legumes, nuts, and seeds, often accompanied by healthy fats such as olive oil and a limited amounts of lean protein from fish or plant-based sources. *Meat is eaten more as a side dish than as a main course.* These diets also incorporate herbs and spices that add both flavor and anti-inflammatory benefits. These nutrient-dense diets are *high in fiber, antioxidants, and phytonutrients*, which work synergistically to protect against chronic diseases and support optimal health. Beyond the nutrient profile, Eastern diets often include mindful eating practices and a cultural focus on communal meals, further enhancing their holistic benefits.

Since the 1950s, a significant body of scientific literature has explored the relationship between diet, health, and disease, *especially heart disease, stroke, obesity, diabetes, and cancer*. One recurring theme has emerged and has been consistently proven over time: *there are health benefits in avoiding animal proteins and processed foods while increasing the intake of plant-based foods*. It is worth reviewing a few of the proven clinical studies and facts here:

- In the Western world, including the United States, *since the 1920s* there has been a sharp rise in the incidence of the diseases I listed above due to the introduction of highly processed and packaged foods, *often found in boxes, bags, and cans*. Alongside the proliferation of fast-food restaurants, sugary drinks, ready-to-eat meals, and TV dinners, America now faces an epidemic of these *entirely preventable and even reversible* diseases. Alarmingly, now with rapid globalization, the detrimental effects of the Western diet are spreading globally, impacting billions more.
- Studies reveal that, while these diseases have been widespread in Western societies, they are nearly nonexistent or significantly less common in many Eastern societies due to dietary differences. This is changing because of the shift in dietary habits of people in Eastern countries to a Western-style diet with processed and animal-based foods.
- Medical research has shown that when individuals from Eastern countries like India, Japan, and China migrate to the United States and switch to a Western diet of highly processed, calorie-dense foods, the incidence of heart disease, obesity, diabetes, and cancer rises dramatically—*often*

surpassing rates in the general American population. For example, the relative risk of heart disease–related mortality in immigrant Asian Indians in the United States is 20 to 50 percent higher than in other groups. Moreover, they tend to develop heart disease five to ten years earlier than other ethnicities.

- Even without migrating to the United States, when Easterners adopt Western diets in their own homelands, the incidence of these diseases skyrockets. In recent years, dietary shifts in India have contributed to its status as the country with the highest number of diabetes cases in the world.
- The converse is also true. When people transition from Western diets to Eastern and Mediterranean diets, their risk for these diseases decreases rapidly and significantly. Several physicians, including Dr. Dean Ornish and Dr. Caldwell Esselstyn from the Cleveland Clinic, have conducted clinical research trials—documented by coronary angiograms—and have clearly demonstrated that heart blockages can be REVERSED with switching to a plant-based lifestyle, even in patients with severe blockages.
- Several large-scale studies have demonstrated a significantly lower incidence of these diseases among individuals following plant-based diets compared with adherents of Western-style diets. Notable examples include the China-Cornell-Oxford Project, also known as the *China Study*, conducted in 1980s involving 6,500 adults from 65 counties in rural China. This study demonstrated strong correlations between dietary habits and chronic diseases. It found that diets high in animal-based foods were linked to increased risk of conditions like heart disease, diabetes, and certain cancers. Conversely, plant-based diets, rich in whole foods, were associated with improved health outcomes and lower rates of chronic illnesses. *Blue Zones*

research from the early 2000s identified five regions where people live longer, healthier lives primarily due to consuming a plant-based diet, moderate caloric intake, regular physical activity, and community involvement with strong social connections. The *EPIC-Oxford study*, conducted between 1993 and 1999, also highlighted the benefits of an Eastern-style, plant-based diet over a Western diet in a cohort of 65,000 people in the United Kingdom. The *Okinawa Centenarian Study* conducted in Japan in the 1970s showed that, compared with people in Western countries, residents of that island had 80 percent less chance of getting heart disease primarily due to a diet that consists primarily of fresh, whole-food, plant-based food with almost no processed food and only a small amount of fish eaten as a side dish.

When I was growing up in India, it was a land of wholesome, plant-based traditions. India is now facing a health crisis fueled by the rise of Western-style fast food restaurants and packaged foods. In recent years, India has experienced a sharp rise in obesity, diabetes, heart disease, and stroke. This alarming trend is primarily due to a shift away from a traditional diet—rich in lentils, legumes, grains, nuts, seeds, fresh fruits, and vegetables—to a Western-style diet dominated by refined sugar, packaged and ultra-processed foods, and fast-food products. I've seen how this shift to processed diets has led India to become the *number one country globally for diabetes*, accounting for 17 percent of the world's total—a preventable tragedy. Returning to traditional, fiber-rich, freshly cooked, plant-based diets and reducing reliance on fast foods and processed foods can make a critical difference, reclaiming health and vitality for millions across India and the world.

The unfortunate reality is that you no longer need to immigrate to the United States to experience the unhealthy consequences of the American diet. When I think about fast-food chains in America, I can't help but imagine their catchphrase being more honest—perhaps saying instead, "Would you like a heart attack to go with that?"

> By following a whole-food, plant-based diet with no processed food, you can decrease your weight, improve blood sugar levels, control blood pressure better, and decrease cholesterol levels.

Our body is an extraordinary system, capable of incredible feats. It's truly astonishing how it processes, assimilates, and utilizes everything we eat and drink with remarkable precision to fuel cellular metabolism and sustain life. *Yet, we often fail to treat it with the respect it deserves.* We would never expect a factory or machine to produce high-quality results if we fed it poor-quality raw materials, but that's exactly what we do to our bodies every day by consuming a Western diet. Despite this, we expect our bodies to perform at their best.

As we've discussed, science clearly shows that to achieve youthfulness, heal diseases, and live longer, *we must shift to a nutrient-dense, whole-food, plant-based diet with complete elimination of processed foods.* This simple yet powerful change is the foundation for lasting vitality, reversing disease, and staying youthful longer.

First Remove the Weeds

During discussion with my patients about nutrition, I always begin by addressing what to remove from their diet to create lasting health benefits. Just as a garden cannot thrive if it's overrun with weeds or polluted by harmful chemicals, the same principle applies to our bodies. You can water, fertilize, and tend to the soil all you want, but if the foundation is compromised, nothing will grow to its full potential. That's why it's crucial to focus not only on what we put into our bodies but also on what we avoid. In my experience, eliminating harmful foods and toxins is often more impactful than simply adding healthy nutrients.

The Unholy Trinity: What to Avoid

Over these years of helping people—including famous personalities, elite athletes, and top performers from around the world—I've seen the devastating impact of what I call the *unholy trinity*: *smoking, alcohol, and poor dietary choices*. And, until you shun these, anything to increase your youthfulness, health, and longevity is just waste of your time, effort, and money. No matter how much money someone has or how many advanced treatments they seek, if these three issues aren't addressed, everything else you do to improve health is just a Band-Aid over a deeper wound. I've seen firsthand how these habits derail not just physical performance but also the aging process itself.

Let's talk about *smoking*. Time and time again, I've witnessed the profound damage smoking does to the body. It's not just a bad habit; chemicals in smoking accelerates cellular dysfunction, blockage of arteries, and aging in otherwise healthy body. Patients who smoked often presented with severe atherosclerosis, heart disease, lung problems, cancers, and premature aging of the whole body. Their muscles didn't recover as quickly, their skin lost elasticity, and they were plagued by fatigue. Even the wealthiest—those who could afford the best treatments in the world—could not escape the damage smoking caused. Quitting smoking is, without a doubt, one of the most transformative things you can do for your health. I've seen it happen with my patients; those who quit noticed a dramatic change in their energy, beauty, and overall health.

The same goes for *alcohol* abuse. I've treated individuals who could afford the most expensive longevity programs, but nothing compares to completely avoiding this harmful substance. Alcohol, especially in excess, accelerates aging in ways that most people don't even realize until it's too late. It works as a toxic chemical, damaging every cell in your body. It damages the liver; affects the brain, heart, pancreas, and other organs; and even erodes emotional well-being. Several ultra-wealthy patients I worked with had access to every advanced treatment under the sun, but until they addressed their alcohol consumption, their efforts to feel and look younger were futile. Once they committed to stopping or at least cutting back alcohol use, the difference in their physical and emotional health was remarkable.

And then there's the *poor diet*—one of the most overlooked yet crucial components of aging well. I believe strongly that it is more important to focus on what to avoid eating. *Watch everything that goes in your mouth.* This includes all deep-fried foods; processed foods with *high sugar, unhealthy fats, and artificial additives*; calorie-dense packaged foods with high sugar, salt, and oils; junk foods; artificial sweeteners; TV dinners; and fast-food restaurants.

These unhealthy foods can lead to chronic inflammation, metabolic imbalances, mitochondrial dysfunction, and a weakened immune system. Toxins present in our food from *pesticides, antibiotics, chemicals, heavy metals, preservatives, and environmental pollutants* further burden the body, increasing oxidative stress and accelerating aging. I've had wealthy individuals who regularly fly in private chefs and nutritionists, but still fall into the trap of these "tasty toxins": too much sugar, processed foods, yummy additives, and unhealthy fats.

> I strongly advise you to remember this fact—you simply cannot expect any sort of youthfulness and longevity without first removing the toxins of the *unholy trinity*: smoking, poor diet, and alcohol. Watch everything that goes in your mouth. Read the food labels like a detective. How can you ever expect to grow a beautiful garden if it is filled with toxins and weeds?

Because of modern Western foods with toxins and genetic modifications, many people are *sensitive or even allergic to gluten and lactose.*

So, for many individuals, it may also be important to avoid *gluten* (mainly wheat, rye, and barley) and *lactose* from dairy products. These products can cause digestive issues, itching, skin rash, anxiety, or chronic fatigue. So, make sure you avoid those foods, even with a plant-based diet. By avoiding these products, within a few weeks you can notice significant improvement in your symptoms.

I would add here that the public has been misled and left confused about the benefits of different types of diets, *especially regarding fats and oils*. We often hear about "good fats" versus "bad fats"—saturated versus unsaturated—and the virtues of oils like olive and vegetable oil. That discussion is all about when these are in an uncooked state, but we don't consume much raw oils or fats. What's rarely discussed is what happens to these oils when we cook, sauté, or fry food with them, especially once they reach their "smoke point"—the temperature at which a particular oil stops shimmering and starts to smoke. At these high temperatures, oils undergo significant chemical changes that produce harmful compounds and denatures even the "good" oil. For instance, beneficial oils like extra virgin olive oil can become a source of health risks once heated too much, transforming from beneficial to harmful.

As I mentioned, *frying oils past their smoke point generates toxins*. These include a dangerous chemical called acrolein, a known carcinogen, and polycyclic aromatic hydrocarbons (PAHs), which have also been linked to cancer. Other harmful byproducts include aldehydes like 4-hydroxy-trans-2-nonenal (HNE), particularly common when frying with omega-6-rich vegetable oils. As we discussed in detail in chapter 6, ultimately, these chemicals and oxidized fats promote chronic inflammation, a key player in aging, arterial blockages (atherosclerosis), cardiovascular disease, stroke, Alzheimer's, and other diseases associated with aging. Recognizing the risks of high-heat cooking methods highlights the importance of choosing lower-temperature cooking techniques to protect the integrity of oils and support long-term health and vitality.

With my own personal experience as well as in my years of clinical experience, I've observed that the accumulation of toxins in food can silently cause serious cellular dysfunction and sabotage our efforts to achieve youthfulness, vitality, and overall health. *You must watch everything that goes in your mouth.* Yes, unfortunately, this list of toxic things to avoid is long because our food chain *prioritizes profits derived from products with an extended shelf life over our health.* What I've learned after all these years is simple: If you want to truly enhance your health, avoid the *unholy trinity. Eliminating smoking, alcohol, and a poor diet isn't just the first step—it's the foundation.* Without this, anything else you do to improve your health and longevity is a waste of time, energy, and money. I've seen it play out in patients from all walks of life, and the truth is, no one is immune to the impact of these destructive habits.

Make the decision to leave them behind, and everything else will start falling into place.

More about Tasty Toxins in Our Food

Besides cutting out food with too much sugar, tasty additives, and unhealthy fats, eliminating or reducing exposure to the following toxins can lead to significant improvements. Here are some of the main categories of food toxins to watch for:

- **Pesticides:** Common examples include glyphosate (herbicide), chlorpyrifos (insecticide), and atrazine (weed killer). Many pesticides interfere with hormones and potentially contribute to metabolic issues and even cancer.
- **Antibiotics:** Antibiotics like tetracycline, penicillin, and sulfonamides are frequently used in livestock farming. Consuming foods from animals treated with these antibiotics can contribute to antibiotic resistance in humans and disrupt gut health by altering the microbiome.
- **Chemical Additives:** As found in processed foods, additives such as butylated hydroxyanisole (BHA), butylated

hydroxytoluene (BHT), and monosodium glutamate (MSG) can provoke inflammation and hormonal disruption.

- **Heavy Metals:** Metals like mercury, lead, cadmium, and arsenic often enter the food supply through polluted water, soil, or industrial processing. They can cause cognitive decline and other health concerns.
- **Preservatives:** Preservatives such as sodium nitrate and sodium nitrite (found in processed meats) and sodium benzoate and potassium sorbate may help extend shelf life but can increase oxidative stress, accelerating aging and raising the risk of certain cancers.
- **Environmental Pollutants:** Chemicals like bisphenol A (BPA), phthalates, and dioxins infiltrate our food supply through plastic packaging and other environmental sources. They are known endocrine disruptors and may elevate risks for metabolic and reproductive issues.
- **Mycotoxins:** Produced by molds, mycotoxins can contaminate foods like grains, nuts, and coffee. Notable examples include aflatoxin (in peanuts and corn) and ochratoxin (found in grains and wine). Chronic exposure has been linked to liver damage, immune suppression, and cancer.
- **Plastics and Packaging Chemicals:** Beyond BPA, other chemicals in food packaging, such as perfluoroalkyl substances (PFAS), are of concern. Often found in nonstick and stain-resistant coatings of cookware, food containers, and waterproof cloths, PFAS chemicals can disrupt hormones and harm the immune system.
- **Advanced Glycation End Products (AGEs):** AGEs form during high-heat cooking, especially in grilled, fried, or roasted foods. Common sources include processed and barbecued meats. AGEs contribute to inflammation and oxidative stress, accelerating aging and increasing the risk of chronic diseases.

- **Artificial Sweeteners:** Studies have identified artificial sweeteners as problematic. Aspartame (NutraSweet, Equal), acesulfame potassium, sucralose, erythritol (Splenda), and xylitol have been linked to an increased risk of cardiovascular problems, arterial blockages, and stroke. I advise my patients against using any artificial sweeteners.
- **Polycyclic Aromatic Hydrocarbons (PAHs):** These form during the combustion of organic matter, often in high-temperature cooking like grilling or smoking. Known carcinogens, PAHs have been linked to various cancers. Limiting charred meats and smoked foods can reduce exposure.
- **Microplastics and Nanoplastics:** Unfortunately, microplastics and nanoplastics have infiltrated every part of our world and food chain. People are exposed to these through the air, food, and even by absorption through the skin from personal care products. Emerging data suggest that these might be harmful to our health. There is no certain way to remove these from our food, but a few practices can help—*avoiding processed food, using filtered water, avoiding plastic containers, cutting back on bottled water, not using plastic containers in the microwave, and using air filters indoors.*

By understanding and addressing these toxins, we can reduce our body's toxic load and create a foundation for health and youthfulness. I advise my patients to *read the labels of foods they consume as if they were Sherlock Holmes.* I've seen patients experience marked improvements simply by minimizing these hidden risks in their diet. Taking small steps, like opting for organic produce, avoiding processed foods, and choosing safer cooking methods can protect our health and vitality long-term.

Processed and Ultra-Processed Foods

In today's world, processed and ultra-processed foods, *usually sold in bags, cans and packages,* have become a dominant feature in Western diets, and *while they may seem convenient, they're doing more harm than good.* These foods are industrially manufactured products *designed to be hyper-palatable and convenient with a prolonged shelf life, but often contain little to no whole, natural ingredients.* Instead, they're high in refined sugars, modified oils, salt, artificial flavors, preservatives, chemicals, hormones, and emulsifiers.

Processed foods are those that have been altered from their original state—think canned vegetables or frozen dinners that have been modified to last longer or taste better. Ultra-processed foods, however, take it a step further and are far worse for your health. These products undergo extensive modifications, and contain long list of artificial ingredients and additives. In the manufacturing process, they lose most of their natural nutrients. Examples of ultra-processed foods include sugary cereals, soda, fast-food, instant noodles, and packaged snacks like chips and cookies.

Here's the problem: these ultra-processed foods are *full of things that fuel inflammation, mess with your metabolism, and strip away your body's natural defenses.* Over time, they can lead to serious health issues like heart disease, stroke, diabetes, and even cancer. And that's not just speculation—there's a lot of solid science behind it. The sugars, trans fats, salt, and chemicals found in ultra-processed foods may taste great in the moment, but they wreak havoc on your body, especially when eaten regularly. And the worst part? These foods are often empty calories, providing little to no nutritional value.

> Science has been clear for several decades: our food chain is the primary driver of America's chronic diseases, including obesity, diabetes, cardiovascular disease, stroke, mood disorders, and cancer. It's as if we've been conducting a century-long chemistry experiment on living human beings—with devastating results.

The good news is that spotting these foods can be pretty easy. *If the ingredient list reads like a chemistry experiment*—filled with long, hard-to-pronounce additives like high-fructose corn syrup or artificial dyes—it's probably ultra-processed. Foods that are packaged, premade, and designed to be super convenient, like chips, energy drinks, or ready-to-eat snacks, often fall into this category. And don't forget about those "hyper-palatable" foods—those irresistible combinations of fat, sugar, and salt that make you want to eat the whole bag. Yep, they're engineered to be addictive.

So how do you avoid these food traps? The answer is simple: stick to whole, fresh foods. *Make fresh fruits and vegetables, whole grains, nuts, seeds, and high fiber the foundation of your meals.* When you do need something packaged, keep it as close to nature as possible—choose items with short ingredient lists made up of things you recognize. *Cooking at home* is a powerful way to take back control, letting you skip the hidden sugars and chemicals that sneak into premade meals. You don't need to be perfect; every small effort has cumulative benefit over time. So, *making even small shifts away from processed foods and toxins can have a huge impact on your long-term health and energy.*

> Returning to a whole-food, fiber-rich, freshly cooked, plant-based diet and reducing reliance on fast foods and processed foods can make a critical difference, reclaiming health and vitality for millions across the world.

Diseases of Abundance

Diseases of abundance—such as *obesity, type 2 diabetes, hypertension, and heart disease*—have become almost synonymous with modern American life and are critical barriers to achieving longevity and an extended healthspan. In my years of practice, I've seen how *easy access to calorie-dense, processed foods and a sedentary lifestyle* contributes to these chronic conditions, which, left unchecked, significantly shorten not only lifespan but the number of years lived in good health. These diseases are often preventable and manageable through lifestyle changes, yet they accumulate over time, leading to complex health issues that drain both personal energy and our resources.

What's promising, though, is that we do have powerful tools for addressing these conditions and promoting longevity. While there are many reasons behind these diseases—from the prevalence of processed foods to the fast pace of modern life—reclaiming control through fresh, nutrient-dense food, moderate eating, and semi-fasting gives us a path to better health.

Low-Calorie Diet

Now let me share some of the tremendous health benefits I've seen with a low-calorie diet. In clinical as well as lab research, so far only *one* thing has passed scientific rigor and has been shown to extend life—and it is *eating less*. Over the years, I've witnessed how reducing calorie intake, even by a modest amount, can lead to remarkable improvements in both health and vitality. People who adopt a low-calorie diet tend to experience better healthspan, enhanced metabolic health, better blood sugar control, and reduced inflammation—all of which are crucial for preventing chronic diseases like obesity, heart disease, and diabetes. I've seen patients not only control diseases better but also report higher energy levels, improved focus, and even better sleep. What I find most encouraging is the simplicity of this approach: small, strategic changes can yield profound and lasting benefits.

A low-calorie diet involves reducing your daily caloric intake by about 20 to 30 percent while ensuring your body gets essential nutrients. This isn't about starvation but about *eating smarter.* Research shows that calorie restriction reduces oxidative stress, minimizes cellular damage, and slows aging. Studies in animals demonstrate *lifespan extensions of up to 40 percent,* and similar mechanisms, like reduced inflammation and enhanced cellular repair, are likely at work in humans.

> In clinical as well as lab research, so far only *one* thing has passed scientific rigor and shown to extend life—it is *eating less calories.*

One striking example comes from a 2013 study in *Diabetes Care*. Researchers found that patients following a calorie-restricted diet achieved better blood sugar control than those undergoing gastric bypass surgery. Another study in 2018 confirmed these findings, emphasizing that calorie restriction alone can deliver significant health improvements—without the risks of invasive surgery.

The goal of a low-calorie diet isn't just to add more years to life but to enhance the quality of those years. By focusing on nutrient-dense foods like vegetables, fruits, whole grains, and lean proteins, you improve blood sugar control, heart health, and cholesterol levels, reducing the time spent managing chronic illnesses. This thoughtful approach isn't about extreme restrictions but about providing your body the fuel it needs for a longer, healthier, and more vibrant life.

Semi-Fasting

Semi-fasting, also known as *intermittent fasting*, is a practice where you cycle between periods of eating and fasting. Semi-fasting is not about drastically cutting calories every day, but rather about controlling *when* you eat. A common method is the *16:8 approach*, where you fast for sixteen hours and eat within an eight-hour window. Some people follow a *5:2 approach*, where they eat normally five days of the week and significantly reduce calories for two days (say, on Mondays and Wednesdays). After some time, you can even use both strategies together to get the maximum benefit from intermittent fasting. The idea is to give your body extended breaks from eating, allowing it to repair, detoxify, and function more efficiently.

During fasting, the body burns stored fat for energy, reduces insulin levels, and initiates autophagy—a process that clears out damaged cells and promotes regeneration. This improves cellular repair, reduces inflammation, and protects against chronic diseases and aging. Research shows that intermittent fasting enhances insulin sensitivity, regulates blood sugar, lowers blood pressure and cholesterol, and boosts brain health by increasing brain-derived neurotrophic factor (BDNF), which supports cognitive function and protects against neurodegeneration. Animal studies even suggest it may extend lifespan by reducing oxidative stress and enhancing cellular efficiency.

> Eating fewer calories without sacrificing nutrition, combined with the strategic use of semi-fasting, leads to improved mitochondrial and metabolic health, better insulin sensitivity, and enhanced energy levels.

Plant-Based Diet: Proven Health Benefits

At this point during my consultation, patients always ask me, "Doc, so what do I eat then?" I start by saying that I have yet to see any *vegetables-and-fruits-only diet* obese person. Then I share that I have personally experienced the transformative power of plant-based diet—a cornerstone of Blue Zone regions. This diet focusses on consuming foods primarily from plants, including fresh fruits and vegetables, whole grains, nuts, legumes, and seeds. Just like me, by *embracing a diverse range of fresh foods in a plant-based diet*, you too can reduce the risk of chronic illnesses and boost your overall vitality.

A plant-based diet is consistently recognized as one of the most effective ways to promote healthspan, increase lifespan, and maintain youthful energy. As we discussed earlier in this chapter, numerous studies back this up, showing that diets rich in fruits, vegetables, whole grains, legumes, nuts, and seeds are associated with *lower risks of chronic diseases like heart disease, diabetes, and certain cancers.* Furthermore, plant-based eating has been shown to improve insulin sensitivity, reduce inflammation, reverse diseases, and enhance overall well-being.

Start caring for your health at the grocery store. I simply don't waste money on buying anything that I know I should not be putting in my mouth. I keep my kitchen clear of all packaged, processed, and ultra-processed foods. I start by filling my kitchen with fresh, colorful whole foods with high fibers and experimenting with new recipes that excite my taste buds. I have learned to read all nutrition labels like a detective, uncovering hidden processed ingredients and their unhealthy counterparts. Soon, I find myself feeling more energized and vibrant. I know that with each delicious, nutritious meal, I'm not just feeding my body, *but also nourishing my future self.*

A word of caution here: remember, everything that is "plant-based" is not necessarily healthy. *Plant-based milk*, like oat milk, almond milk, and soy milk, are ultra-processed and best to avoid. *French fries and Oreo cookies* may be free from animal products, but they're loaded with unhealthy fats, refined sugars, and processed ingredients that offer little to no nutritional value. These foods are prime examples of *empty calories*, providing too many calories without the essential nutrients our cells need to function optimally. In fact, as we discussed, these ultra-processed plant-based foods can do more harm than good, contributing to inflammation, weight gain, and other health issues. True health comes from whole, minimally processed foods that fuel our bodies, not just fill them.

High-Fiber Content in Plant-Based Diet

Increasingly, it is becoming clear that dietary fiber is one of the simplest yet most powerful ways to support health and slow the aging process. Fiber, *primarily found in plant-based foods*, plays a vital role in supporting digestion, maintaining a balanced gut microbiome, and stabilizing blood sugar levels—all essential factors for longevity and overall vitality. From leafy greens to legumes, a plant-based diet naturally provides high levels of fiber that contribute to better health outcomes and an extended healthspan.

One of the greatest benefits of fiber is its impact on gut health. These are not just some bulking agents for your gut. *With these fibers, you are actually feeding your good microbiome*, which is so essential for your health and disease management. Fiber acts as a prebiotic, feeding beneficial bacteria in the gut that support immunity, improve digestion, and help to reduce inflammation. We know chronic, low-grade inflammation is a key driver of aging and age-related diseases, and by nourishing the gut microbiome, *fiber helps lower this inflammation*, creating a foundation for long-term health.

In addition to gut health, fiber has a profound effect on blood sugar regulation and cardiovascular health. By slowing the absorption of sugars, fiber helps prevent spikes in blood glucose and insulin, which can *protect against insulin resistance*—a common risk factor for metabolic diseases like diabetes and a driver of accelerated aging. *Soluble fibers*, such as those found in oats, beans, apples, chia, flaxseeds, and psyllium can also bind to cholesterol in the digestive system, helping to lower LDL cholesterol levels and reduce the risk of cardiovascular disease.

I read a recent research paper about beneficial effects of *hemp prebiotic fiber*, which is said to contain two bioactive compounds that encourage the growth of a good microbiome in the gut. Hemp and marijuana plants are both the same species, but hemp contains almost negligible amounts of *THC* (*tetrahydrocannabinol*), a psychoactive chemical. I do not recommend hemp fiber as yet; I mention this here only as interesting information and to keep an eye on this research as it evolves.

What makes fiber so beneficial is how easily accessible it is through a whole-food, plant-based diet. By simply including more fresh fruits and vegetables, whole grains, nuts, and legumes in daily meals, it becomes easy to reach optimal fiber levels without supplements. Fiber from whole foods also provides a host of other age-supporting nutrients like antioxidants, vitamins, and minerals, further enhancing the body's defenses against oxidative stress, cellular damage, and the visible signs of aging.

Blue Zone Diet

One powerful example that highlights the benefits of a plant-based diet is the Blue Zone diet, which is practiced in regions known for their exceptional longevity. As we have discussed previously, the Blue Zones—Ikaria (Greece), Okinawa (Japan), Sardinia (Italy), Nicoya (Costa Rica), and Loma Linda (California)—are areas where people live significantly longer, often reaching one hundred years of age or more. A common factor among these regions is their *predominantly plant-based diets, which emphasize vegetables, legumes, fruits, whole grains, and healthy fats like olive oil, while meat and processed foods are consumed in minimal amounts.*

> The success of Blue Zones populations of centenarians provides living proof that a diet centered on plants not only extends life but ensures that those extra years are spent in good health.

In these Blue Zones, people are not just living longer—they're living better. Their plant-based diets provide the foundation for a long healthspan—the number of years they live in good health, free from chronic disease and frailty. These diets are nutrient-dense and anti-inflammatory, helping to protect against oxidative stress, regulate blood sugar levels, and maintain heart and brain health. The high fiber content in these diets also supports gut health, which is increasingly recognized as a key player in overall well-being and aging.

Proven Benefits of a Plant-Based Diet

The plant-based diet has gained widespread attention for its health benefits, many of which are backed by robust scientific research. Let us now explore the proven benefits of a plant-based diet, supported by scientific studies.

Longevity and Youthful Energy: Research consistently demonstrates that a plant-based diet is strongly associated with increased life expectancy and healthspan. A plant-based diet has shown to *increase telomere length*, signifying longevity. A comprehensive study from Harvard University found that diets rich in whole plant foods significantly reduce the risk of premature death from causes such as *heart disease, cancer, and diabetes*. These foods help *reduce inflammation and protect against cellular damage caused by oxidative stress*, which accelerates aging and increases the risk of age-related diseases.

Chronic Inflammation: A healthy diet is a major determinant of our inflammatory state, and inflammation is now widely regarded as the common denominator in nearly every major disease. A plant-based diet has been shown to reduce inflammation in the body. Plant-based foods are rich in antioxidants and phytonutrients, which combat oxidative stress and lower levels of inflammatory biomarkers. Moreover, a plant-based diet minimizes pro-inflammatory processed foods, further enhancing healthspan and supporting conditions linked to chronic inflammation, such as lupus, rheumatoid arthritis, chronic fatigue syndrome, heart disease, diabetes, and arthritis. It's an excellent way to nourish your body while keeping inflammation in check.

Insulin Sensitivity and Metabolic Health: One of the most important areas where plant-based diets excel is in improving insulin sensitivity and preventing insulin resistance—a key driver of type 2 diabetes and *metabolic syndrome* (combination of obesity, low good cholesterol, and high blood pressure, fats, and sugar). Diets high in fiber from plant foods help stabilize blood sugar levels, reduce insulin spikes, and improve overall metabolic function.

This has been backed by a tremendous amount of clinical research, including a study published in the medical journal *Diabetes Care*, which found that individuals who followed a plant-based diet had a 34 percent lower risk of developing type 2 diabetes. The *low glycemic load of a plant-based diet with high fiber* content helps maintain steady blood sugar levels, keeping energy levels stable throughout the day and preventing the energy crashes often associated with high-sugar, processed diets. This not only enhances your energy but also reduces the risk of developing insulin resistance.

Both the American and Canadian Diabetes Associations recognize the benefits of vegetarian (a plant-based diet that includes dairy and honey) and vegan (a strict plant-based diet that excludes even dairy and honey) eating patterns. These diets have been shown to improve glycemic control, body weight, and cardiovascular risk factors. Additionally, the American College of Endocrinologists—experts in diabetes care—advocates for a plant-based diet as a vital component of managing type 2 diabetes.

Heart Health: One of the most significant benefits of a plant-based diet is its positive impact on cardiovascular health. Studies have shown that plant-based diets can reduce the risk of and even reverse heart disease by lowering blood pressure, reducing LDL (bad) cholesterol, and improving overall heart function. In fact, research from the American Heart Association suggests that people who consume more plant-based foods and fewer animal products *have a lower risk of heart attacks and strokes.* This is primarily because plant-based diets are so rich in fiber, antioxidants, and healthy fats, all of which contribute to better heart health.

Reduced Risk of Chronic Diseases and Cancers: A plant-based diet has been shown to reduce the risk of developing several chronic diseases, including type 2 diabetes, obesity, and certain cancers. Studies also link a higher intake of plant foods with a *lower risk of colorectal, breast, and prostate cancers*. This is due to the *anti-inflammatory and antioxidant* properties of fruits, vegetables, and whole grains, which help protect cells from oxidative damage.

Weight Management: Contrary to popular wisdom, I believe the key to sustainable weight loss lies not in forcing your metabolism but in reducing inflammation in your body. Plant-based diets help lower inflammation and are rich in fiber, making them highly effective for weight management. They are also naturally lower in calories, which further supports healthy weight loss. Research shows that individuals who follow plant-based eating patterns, *especially when combined with intermittent fasting*, tend to have a lower body mass index (BMI) compared to those who consume a diet high in animal products. The fiber in plants helps you feel fuller for longer, reduces overeating, and improves digestion, leading to healthier weight maintenance over time.

Improved Gut Health: The high fiber content of plant-based diets promotes a healthy gut microbiome. Fiber serves as food for beneficial gut bacteria, supporting digestion and enhancing immune function. As we have discussed previously, a healthy microbiome plays a crucial role in helping with auto-immune diseases, preventing gastrointestinal disorders, reducing inflammation, and even improving mental health. Studies suggest that plant-based diets *increase the diversity of beneficial gut bacteria*, which is linked to better overall health.

Mental Health: I believe many people underestimate the profound impact diet has on mental health. Research shows that diets high in ultra-processed foods are strongly associated with an increased risk of mental illnesses like depression and anxiety. For instance, a 2024 study published in the British Medical Journal found that consuming ultra-processed foods increased the risk of depression by 22% and anxiety by 48%. But the good news is that the reverse is also true. A review of 13 studies, published in Nutrition Reviews in early 2025, revealed that plant-based diets, such as the Mediterranean diet, can significantly decrease the risk of depression, anxiety, and even attention deficit hyperactivity disorder (ADHD). Additionally, a 2024 study of 7,434 adults demonstrated that incorporating more legumes, vegetables, fruits, yogurt, and seafood into one's diet helps lower stress levels.

Environmental and Ethical Benefits: While the health benefits of a plant-based diet are significant, it's also worth noting the positive environmental and ethical impacts. A plant-based diet is often linked to sustainable living, helping to preserve the planet for future generations.

The science is clear: a plant-based diet is one of the best ways to support longevity, healthspan, and overall vitality. The success of Blue Zone populations provides living proof that a diet centered on plants not only extends life but ensures that those extra years are spent in good health. Whether it's improving insulin sensitivity, reducing inflammation, or promoting youthful energy, the plant-based approach offers a comprehensive strategy for aging gracefully while maintaining a high quality of life. By embracing this way of eating, you are investing in your long-term health and setting the stage for a longer, healthier, and more vibrant future.

Fact: Eating Is a Learned Behavior and Can Be Unlearned

Let me remind you of this key fact: eating is far more than a biological necessity—*it's a learned behavior shaped by culture, upbringing, and personal experiences.* It is estimated that 1.5 billion people—approximately 22 percent of the world's population—have never eaten meat, and they're perfectly fine with it. However, I'm not sure the same can be said about processed food.

From childhood, we are taught what to eat, how to eat, and even why we eat. These lessons can come from family traditions, social norms, and emotional cues—like being rewarded with sweets for good behavior or turning to comfort foods in times of stress. Over time, *these learned patterns become automatic, creating habits that feel as natural as hunger itself.*

In America our eating habits are deeply rooted in a *culture of convenience and hurrying,* where processed and packaged foods dominate the shelves and dinner tables. From childhood, many are taught to reach for boxed cereals, frozen dinners, or drive-through meals—*quick fixes that prioritize speed over nutrition.* Ultimately, these ultra-processed foods *rewire taste buds*, making the bold flavors of salt, sugar, and fat feel irresistible while the natural sweetness of a ripe fruit or the subtle bitterness of greens becomes less appealing or is completely forgotten by the brain.

But here's the empowering fact: these preferences are not fixed. Just as eating habits are learned, they can also be unlearned. The brain's remarkable neuroplasticity allows us to break old habits and establish new, healthier ones. For example, research has shown that repeated exposure can reshape our preferences; nutritious yet unfamiliar foods can become as appealing as the yummy junk foods we once craved.

Just as eating a processed and animal-based American diet is a learned behavior, transitioning to a whole-food, plant-based diet with zero processed food is entirely possible. The brain and palate can adapt. Studies show that with consistent exposure to whole foods, our taste buds recalibrate, finding pleasure in the richness of natural, unprocessed ingredients. But this retraining of our taste buds demands a clear understanding of its importance and an unwavering commitment to the process.

So How Do I Really Unlearn a Lifelong Behavior, You Ask

Remember, *every small step rewires your brain*, paving the way for a healthier relationship with food. The foods you eat today don't have to define you forever. With practice, you can unlearn what doesn't serve you and rediscover the joy of eating to thrive. Here are few tips to switching to this new "plant-based, zero processed food" lifestyle:

Awareness and Intentionality: Unlearning unhealthy eating patterns begins with awareness and intentionality. Shifting from a processed diet to a whole-food, plant-based lifestyle starts with small, intentional changes. Begin by removing the most obvious culprits—soda, packaged snacks, and fast food—and replacing them with whole, nutrient-dense alternatives like fresh fruits, nuts, or roasted vegetables. Plan your meals around whole grains, legumes, and vibrant produce, letting their natural flavors take center stage.

Triggers: Identifying the triggers behind your food choices—are you eating because you're hungry, bored, or seeking comfort? Understanding these motivations allows you to interrupt the cycle and make more conscious decisions.

Favor Consistency over Perfection: Gradually replace old habits with new rituals, like savoring a piece of fruit instead of reaching for a sugary snack.

Mindfulness: Mindful eating can be transformative in this transition. Slow down, savor the taste of real food, and notice how your body feels when nourished by wholesome ingredients. Over time, the addictive pull of processed foods fades as your body and mind begin to crave the vitality of plant-based meals.

Reframing Mind: Studies also suggest that reframing how you think about food—viewing it as nourishment for the body and mind rather than a source of indulgence—can create lasting change.

Enjoy New Frontiers: To succeed, embrace the journey as an exploration of new flavors and possibilities—experiment with spices, discover global cuisines, and build a deeper connection with the food that fuels you. The shift might feel challenging at first, but every meal is an opportunity to unlearn the processed habits of the past and step into a more vibrant, healthful way of eating.

An "All-You-Can-Eat" Diet: Simple Tips to Embrace a Plant-Based Lifestyle

I grew up in India as a vegetarian but adopted an American diet almost thirty-five years ago when I immigrated here. It was not as difficult for me to switch back to a plant-based diet. I understand that for most Americans who grew up here, switching entirely to a whole-food, plant-based diet is extremely challenging—especially for those who have eaten meat their entire lives, given the available food options in America and the demands of our busy lifestyles. So, in my practice, I advise my patients that, during the transition, it is best to make sensible choices, avoid eating mammals, and take only fresh seafood and lean organic chicken and turkey that is baked, grilled, or sliced. But remember, most of the meat we consume is processed—unless you fish, hunt for your own food, or purchase it at fresh food markets

Start with the basics: fresh fruits, vegetables, whole grains (oats, barley, rice, wheat, teff, millet, rye), legumes (including beans, peas, lentils, chickpeas, peanuts, and soybeans), and lightly cooked meals—think *slow-cooked stews*, and even recipes for *"five-minute" fresh meals*. Incorporating tea, seeds (such as chia, sunflower, and flaxseed) and nuts (including almonds, walnuts, and cashews) into your diet further boosts fiber and nutrient levels while offering comfort and ease in daily meals.

Transitioning to a plant-based diet may feel daunting, *so take it gradually*. I often tell my patients to *start with just two or three days a week* focused on plant-based meals or *even just one meal a day*. Small steps—whether it's switching your breakfast to a fiber-rich smoothie or making lunch a hearty vegetable soup—lay the foundation for lasting change. In the beginning, if you feel the need for animal protein, consider adding mildly grilled or baked poultry and seafood, rather than mammal meat (such as pork and beef). Over time, this gradual shift can make the benefits of a fully plant-based diet more accessible and sustainable.

Foods to Avoid

- *All* animal products, including but not limited to, mammals, birds, fish, seafood, eggs, dairy, reptiles, amphibians, and insects.
- Foods with toxins, as listed above.
- If sensitive, gluten (mainly wheat, rye, and barley) and lactose from dairy products.
- Ultra-processed foods.
- Fried foods, especially deep-fried foods.
- Soda, carbonated drinks, and watch for those "healthy drinks"—many contain high sugar, sweeteners, and toxins.
- Calorie-dense foods such as candies, nut butters, energy bars, pastries, cakes, pizza, and fried foods.
- Packaged and canned foods with high amounts of refined sugar and salt, and unhealthy and fried oils (junk foods, TV dinners, microwavable foods stored in the cabinet).
- Fast-food restaurants.
- All artificial sweeteners; use honey, maple syrup, or dates instead.

Key Tips to Healthy Eating

- As we discussed, remember that what you love to eat is a learned behavior and can be unlearned. But have patience! It takes time to unlearn lifelong habits.
- Focus on consistency more than perfection. Every small change adds up to huge results over time.
- No need to count calories with a plant-based lifestyle.
- Slowly switch to a whole-food, plant-based diet—start with one meal a day or just one to two days a week.
- Read food labels like a detective.
- Only buy healthy foods to eat.
- Plan your meals instead of grabbing something to eat at the last minute. This is especially important if you work outside the home.
- Before your main meal, eat fiber-rich foods such as fresh vegetables as salads.
- Consider intermittent fasting.
- A plant-based diet provides enough proteins for most, but you can add protein powders such as those from pea, chia, flaxseeds.
- Learn to cook more at home as much as possible.
- Consume homemade fresh smoothies with fresh fruits and vegetables.
- If you must eat meat, especially during the transition, eat it as a side dish and not as your main course. Avoid eating mammals and take only fresh seafood and lean organic chicken and turkey that is baked, grilled, or sliced.
- Take extra omega-3 from chia seeds and flaxseeds.
- Take supplements, especially a multivitamin with B_{12} and folate, Vitamin D_3, and magnesium. Premenopausal females may need liquid iron supplementation.

- Here are a few good resources to learn more about this new lifestyle: https://omdfortheplanet.com, https://www.forksoverknives.com, https://nutritionfacts.org.

These simple shifts are foundational in transforming health and longevity. For years, I've guided patients toward these habits and seen dramatic benefits in vitality, energy, and resilience. Now I'd like to share *my personal simple recipes for three smoothies* that I've been using for years, each offering enormous health benefits:

Wellness Drink: Instead of purchasing wellness drinks or shots from stores, here's what I do: Blend a few oranges with ginger, lemon, turmeric, black pepper, mint, and honey. Adjust the amounts to your taste and enjoy this refreshing, real wellness drink.

Morning Smoothie: I am so grateful that I have an old orange tree in my backyard that still gives me plenty of fresh oranges, almost all year long. Most mornings, I start my day with a blend of oranges, blueberries, strawberries, banana, chia seeds, cinnamon, and pea protein powder with L-leucine, turmeric, creatine, and urolithin A. It's the perfect wake-me-up energy health drink.

Afternoon Green Detox Smoothie: For a great anti-inflammatory boost and gut microbiome support, blend apples, pineapple, ginger, spinach or kale, mint, turmeric, and triphala herbal mix. This drink is as detoxifying as it is rejuvenating.

Doc, Do I Really Need to Change My Diet?

"Come to the edge," he said.
"We can't, we're afraid!" they responded.
"Come to the edge," he said.
"We can't, we will fall!" they responded.
"Come to the edge," he said.
And so they came.
And he pushed them.
And they flew.
—Guillaume Apollinaire, French poet

I hear this question from my patients all the time: *"Do I really need to change my diet?"* My answer is always the same: absolutely, *yes*. If you're at all serious about being healthy, living longer, and preventing or even reversing chronic diseases, changing your diet is sacred. *Switching to a plant-based diet is like investing in your very own future self.* Now you even have the know-how needed to make this transition.

You see, science has been clear for several decades: our food chain is the primary driver of America's chronic diseases, including obesity, diabetes, cardiovascular disease, stroke, mood disorders, and cancer. It's as if we've been running a chemistry experiment on living human beings for nearly a century, with horrible results.

I often challenge my patients—half jokingly but with complete sincerity—with a "money-back guarantee." If you've followed all the advice from your physicians so far, yet you still struggle to manage your chronic diseases, feel tired, weak, and depleted, or experience shortness of breath after a short walk, then here's my challenge for you: *Make just ONE change. Switch to a fresh, whole-food, plant-based diet with absolutely no processed food for six weeks.* No exceptions, no cheating. Commit fully. And I promise you'll begin to see remarkable improvements—not just in how you feel, but also in controlling your blood sugar, blood pressure, cholesterol levels, and overall health. You really have nothing to lose.

As a physician and healer, I have to be perfectly candid: I find it absolutely appalling how the American food chain is overwhelmingly dominated by processed products—*packaged in bags, boxes, or cans.* From the seeds to the farming practices, manufacturing techniques, and packaging, every step of this process is designed with one goal: *extending shelf life for financial gain and catering to the convenience of our rushed lifestyles.*

No matter how persuasive the advertisements or enticing the labels may seem, this so-called food is not designed with your health in mind. It's inundated with genetic engineering, pesticides, chemicals, preservatives, antibiotics, ultra-processing, and who knows what else.

America excels in so many ways—but it also has a unique talent for taking a fresh, wholesome potato and transforming it into a salty, fatty, and highly addictive bag of yummy potato chips that can last for months to years. *Packed with "tasty toxins," these chips offer absolutely no nutritional value.* What they do provide, however, is a surefire way to gain weight, raise your blood pressure, increase your cholesterol, and set yourself up for diabetes, heart attacks, strokes, and potentially even cancer and depression.

Let's be honest: Have you ever stopped at eating just a few chips without finishing the whole bag? Most of us grew up with this crunchy, addictive taste—how wonderful, right? Or is it?

We pour immense time, money, and effort into "fixing" these diseases AFTER they're diagnosed, yet do almost nothing to prevent them in the first place. The time has come for all of us, as consumers, to take back control of our health and safeguard ourselves against these preventable conditions.

> **A Challenge to All Readers:**
> **You've Got Nothing to Lose**
>
> So far, if you've been doing everything you've been told by your physicians, but still struggle to manage your weight, diabetes, hypertension, and high cholesterol levels, despite taking all your medicines; or if you are still suffering from any of the symptoms, such as low energy, brain fog, weight gain, chest pain, depression, anxiety, or shortness of breath, then I have a challenge for you. *Commit to just one change: switch to a fresh, whole-food, plant-based diet with NO processed food for six weeks.* No cheating. Stick with it, and I know, you'll start to notice significant improvements—not just in how you feel, but in managing your blood sugar, blood pressure, cholesterol levels, and overall health. You can thank me later.

Of course, we all want to stay healthy, live longer, and prevent or reverse disease. As the great philosopher Bob Dylan once sang, "The answer, my friend, is blowin' in the wind." The solution lies in adopting a diet that includes absolutely *ZERO* processed food and is primarily fresh, whole-food, and plant-based, with little to no lean meat.

Let me be clear: Based on an abundance of scientific evidence, I strongly advise eliminating both processed food and meat from your diet. However, if you must prioritize, cutting out all processed food is far more critical than eliminating meat. It's worth noting that nearly all the meat we consume is processed unless you fish or hunt it yourself. My advice to anyone ready to take control of their health: *stop eating processed food immediately.*

Is it easy to do? Absolutely not. Can it be done? YES, it absolutely can. We all know so well—*Nothing great in life comes easy.* Like any important project in life, it requires clear goals, an *"I'm all in"* commitment, grit, hard work, and persistence. And don't worry if you slip—because you will. We all do. When that happens, I always find comfort in this simple yet profound Chinese proverb: *Fall seven times, get up eight.* Stay the course and remember that it takes time to unlearn a lifelong behavior. Patience is key. As Warren Buffett wisely said, "No matter how great the talent or effort, some things just take time: you can't produce a baby in one month by getting nine women pregnant."

A Note on Ozempic

GLP-1 (glucagon-like peptide-1) agonist drugs, such as Ozempic (semaglutide) and liraglutide are used for weight loss and are all over the news these days. GLP-1 is a hormone primarily produced in the gut that plays a significant role in regulating blood sugar levels, promoting satiety (the feeling of fullness), and enhancing insulin sensitivity. GLP-1 agonist drugs such as Ozempic have been developed to mimic this hormone's effects and are now commonly used to help manage type 2 diabetes and, increasingly, to support weight loss. These drugs work by slowing stomach emptying, increasing insulin production, and reducing appetite, leading to better blood sugar control and potential weight management benefits. While these GLP-1 drugs are helpful for many patients, *they are not risk-free, especially when used long-term.* It is a good idea to help your body make this hormone naturally. There are ways to naturally support and enhance GLP-1 levels in the body.

How to Increase GLP-1 Naturally

Natural methods to boost GLP-1 primarily revolve around diet and lifestyle choices that encourage the body's own production of this hormone. Incorporating higher levels of fiber, healthy fats, and polyphenols—compounds found in colorful fruits and vegetables—can stimulate GLP-1 secretion and enhance its benefits. Physical activity, particularly aerobic exercise, has also been shown to increase GLP-1 levels, further supporting metabolism and blood sugar balance.

Foods That Stimulate GLP-1 (That's Good!)

- **Herbs:** Certain herbs, such as berberine, tea, curcumin, cinnamon, resveratrol, ginseng, and gardenia, can boost GLP-1 release.
- **Supplements:** Few supplements such as magnesium, vitamin D_3, and chromium can help boost GLP-1 levels.
- **High-Fiber Foods:** Foods rich in soluble fiber, such as oats, legumes, and flaxseeds help slow digestion and promote GLP-1 secretion.
- **Omega-3 Fatty Acids:** Found in chia seeds, walnuts, cashews, and flaxseeds, omega-3s have been shown to support GLP-1 production.
- **Fruits and Vegetables:** Apples, citrus fruits, berries, and leafy greens contain antioxidants and fiber that enhance GLP-1 release.
- **Fermented Foods:** Foods like yogurt, kefir, and kimchi support a healthy gut microbiome, which can positively influence GLP-1 levels.
- **Proteins:** Proteins such as plant-based proteins like tofu can also increase GLP-1 secretion, particularly when combined with fiber.

Foods That Inhibit or Reduce GLP-1 (Not Good!)

- **Carrageenan:** Derived from red algae, this a food additive can inhibit GLP-1 secretion.
- **High-Sugar and Refined Carbohydrate Foods:** Foods like pastries, sugary cereals, and sweetened beverages cause rapid spikes and drops in blood sugar, which can disrupt GLP-1 signaling.
- **Highly Processed Foods:** Ultra-processed foods that contain artificial additives, unhealthy fats, and minimal fiber have been associated with reduced GLP-1 response.
- **Saturated and Trans Fats:** High levels of unhealthy fats found in fried and fatty fast foods may interfere with GLP-1 secretion.

By choosing natural ways to stimulate GLP-1—focusing on whole, fiber-rich foods and healthy fats while minimizing processed sugars and unhealthy fats—you can enhance the benefits of this hormone for blood sugar balance, appetite control, and overall metabolic health.

In this chapter, I've laid out some of the key nutritional components of the VitalLife program to achieve optimal healthspan, youthfulness and longevity. I feel compelled to reiterate here that the first step in any wellness and longevity journey is to remove harmful foods and toxins, and reset your body to a cleaner, healthier state. Once you've built that foundation, the next step is focusing on healthy nutrition.

As we move forward, it's time to talk about the other key pillar of health: exercise. Let's explore how a regular exercise routine can amplify the benefits of nutrition and help you give vitality with strength and energy.

CHAPTER 16

Exercise for Strength and Vitality

> Those who think they have no time for exercise will sooner or later have to find time for illness.
> —Edward Stanley, British statesman (1826–1893)

> Exercise is the key not only to physical health but to peace of mind.
> —Nelson Mandela, anti-apartheid activist and first president of South Africa (1918–2013)

As a physician with many years of experience, I've found that most of my patients have already heard the basics from their doctors countless times. You likely already know that regular exercise is essential—especially as you age. It helps preserve muscle mass, maintain bone density, and support overall physical and mental function. But what I've seen firsthand is how exercise goes beyond the physical. It profoundly impacts social connections and emotional well-being, enriching the lives of people from all walks of life.

Rather than diving into the nitty-gritty of exercise routines and techniques, which can be a snooze-fest, I want to focus on the exercises needed to support longevity and combat the dangerous condition known as sarcopenia. We discussed it earlier along with treatment options in chapter 12, where we examine metabolism. In my years of treating patients from all over the world, I've seen the incredible benefits of strength training and other targeted exercises in preventing and reversing sarcopenia, ultimately promoting vitality and adding years to people's lives.

Exercise is often celebrated as the fountain of youth, and for good reason. As we age, muscle mass declines, metabolism slows, and energy levels drop. Yet, regular physical activity can profoundly counteract these effects, helping to boost physical strength, mental clarity, and emotional balance. Whether it's walking, strength training, or yoga, exercise supports overall health, delays the aging process, and promotes longevity.

The studies of centenarians, such as *Blue Zone Project, Okinawa Centenarian Study, and New England Centenarian Study* have shown the role of physical activity. These studies show that longevity is not tied to genetics alone—environmental, lifestyle, and social factors play an even larger role. The centenarians in these regions shared common traits, including strong social connections, regular physical activity, plant-based diets, and an enduring sense of purpose.

At its core, exercise works on a cellular level to rejuvenate the body. Incorporating regular physical activity into your routine is one of the most effective ways to maintain vitality and live a longer, healthier, and more fulfilling life.

I strongly advocate for *exercising outdoors*, particularly in natural surroundings. Whether it's a gentle stroll near your home or workplace, a walk in the park, hiking, running, biking, morning yoga on the beach, swimming, fishing, or even frequenting the zoo, being in the open air offers benefits that indoor spaces simply can't match. Growing up, my family and I would often spend a day at the Delhi zoo, drawn by the fact that it didn't charge an entrance fee at the time. To this day, I personally find a visit to the zoo far more enjoyable than shopping in a mall.

> **Exercising with others can help you avoid the epidemic of loneliness and boost your emotional well-being.**

Exercise Promotes Both Longevity and Healthspan

By embracing a well-rounded exercise routine that includes strength, aerobic, and flexibility training, you can significantly improve both your lifespan and healthspan—ensuring that the years ahead are full of energy, strength, mobility, and emotional well-being. Through its effects on the heart, muscles, brain, and immune system, *exercise doesn't just add years to your life—it adds life to your years.* Some of the key benefits in this regard include:

Cellular Health and Mitochondria: Exercise works on a cellular level, boosting mitochondrial function and increasing the number of mitochondria in cells—essential for energy production and reducing oxidative stress, a major driver of aging. Studies show that regular physical activity can improve cellular repair mechanisms, delaying the aging process and supporting longevity.

Cardiovascular Health: Engaging in regular aerobic exercise, such as walking, running, swimming, or cycling, improves heart health, lowers blood pressure, and reduces the risk of heart disease—the leading cause of death worldwide. Exercise improves circulation, ensuring that all organs receive the oxygen and nutrients they need to function optimally. This not only extends lifespan but enhances your day-to-day vitality.

Muscle Mass and Bone Density: Aging leads to the natural decline of muscle mass, known as sarcopenia, and to a decrease in bone density. Strength training and weight-bearing exercises can prevent and reverse this, keeping muscles strong and bones dense, reducing the risk of falls, fractures, and frailty. Exercise also stimulates the release of hormones that are essential for muscle repair and growth, ensuring that physical function is maintained throughout life.

Brain Health and Cognitive Function: Physical activity plays a significant role in maintaining brain health. Exercise increases the production of brain-derived neurotrophic factor (BDNF), which supports the growth and survival of neurons, enhancing memory and cognitive function. Regular exercise can slow the progression of neurodegenerative diseases like Alzheimer's and reduce the risk of age-related cognitive decline.

Immune Health: The reduction of inflammation through exercise also plays a pivotal role. We discussed how chronic inflammation is a crucial factor in contributing to the development of age-related diseases like diabetes, heart disease, and cancer. Exercise reduces this inflammation, promoting a healthier immune response, which, as we have discussed, supports longevity and a better quality of life.

Emotional Well-Being: In addition to the physical benefits, exercise has a profound beneficial effect on emotional well-being. It *stimulates the production of endorphins*, which elevate mood, reduce stress, and promote a positive mental outlook. Regular physical activity is also linked to better sleep quality, which is essential for both physical health and emotional balance. Numerous studies show that people who exercise consistently experience less anxiety, fewer symptoms of depression, and improved resilience to life's challenges. Exercise can be particularly *effective in reducing chronic stress*, which accelerates the aging process. By lowering cortisol levels and promoting relaxation, activities like yoga, tai chi, and aerobic exercise create a state of balance in both the mind and body, supporting long-term health and vitality.

Building Social Connections: Exercising with others can transform physical activity into a powerful social experience. Whether it's through group fitness classes, walking clubs, or yoga sessions, the shared connection fosters emotional resilience and helps combat loneliness—an issue that becomes especially critical in later years. Staying socially connected is vital, not just for avoiding the *epidemic of loneliness* often seen in older adults, but also for enhancing longevity and extending healthspan. Group activities provide a meaningful way to nurture these connections while supporting both mental and physical well-being.

Types of Exercises for Optimal Aging

- **Strength Training:** Engage in weightlifting, resistance band work, or bodyweight exercises two or three times per week to maintain muscle mass and bone density, which are crucial for preventing sarcopenia and staying physically capable as you age.
- **Aerobic Exercise:** Incorporate walking, swimming, or cycling three to five times a week to boost cardiovascular health, enhance endurance, and maintain a healthy metabolism.
- **Flexibility and Balance:** Practices like yoga and Pilates are essential for improving joint flexibility, balance, and reducing the risk of falls as we age.
- **Mind-Body Exercises:** Activities like tai chi and yoga also promote mindfulness, reduce stress, and improve emotional well-being, making them a vital part of a comprehensive exercise routine for aging well.

Focus on Sarcopenia and Aging: A Multifactorial Challenge

As we explored in depth in chapter 12, sarcopenia—the loss of muscle mass and strength—is a significant driver of the aging process. Preventing and treating sarcopenia is essential for any effective longevity program. It also serves as a cornerstone of the Vital-Life program, as highlighted in an earlier chapter. In this section,

I'll shift the focus to the exercises that play a crucial role in combating and managing sarcopenia.

Prevent and Alleviate Sarcopenia with These Exercises

To prevent and improve age-related sarcopenia, incorporating a well-rounded exercise regimen focused on strength training, aerobic exercise, and flexibility/balance exercises is key. Below are specific types of exercises recommended to address sarcopenia:

Strength Training (Resistance Exercises):

The most effective way to prevent and reverse sarcopenia is through resistance training, which includes activities like weightlifting, bodyweight exercises, and resistance band workouts. This type of training strengthens muscles and enhances muscle mass and bone density by applying resistance. Research shows that even older adults can significantly increase muscle mass and strength with consistent resistance training. Additionally, it boosts mitochondrial number and function in muscles, which helps metabolism, insulin resistance, and chronic inflammation. It also elevates levels of key muscle-building hormones, such as IGF-1, which are essential for maintaining muscle quality and function.

- **Weightlifting:** Exercises like squats, deadlifts, bench presses, and leg presses are highly effective for building lower body and upper body strength.
- **Bodyweight Exercises:** Exercises such as pushups, squats, lunges, and planks are excellent for those who may not have access to equipment.
- **Resistance Bands:** These are a low-impact and travel-friendly option, perfect for enhancing muscle tone and building strength. Exercises like banded rows, leg curls, and chest presses can help target different muscle groups.

- **Machines:** Strength-training machines found in most gyms (for instance, leg press, lat pull-downs, chest press) offer a safe and controlled way to build muscle mass and strength, especially for beginners.
  Frequency: Engage in strength training two or three times per week, being sure to target all major muscle groups.

Aerobic Exercise

While resistance training is vital for building muscle, aerobic exercise helps improve cardiovascular health, endurance, and blood flow to muscles. Aerobic exercises can help maintain endurance and mobility, allowing older adults to stay active for longer.

- **Walking:** A low-impact, simple way to improve endurance and circulation. Aim for thirty to forty-five minutes of brisk walking, five days a week.
- **Cycling:** Either outdoors or on a stationary bike, cycling strengthens leg muscles and improves cardiovascular health.
- **Swimming:** This full-body workout is gentle on the joints while still building endurance and supporting muscle strength.
- **Dancing or Low-Impact Aerobics Classes:** Great for improving cardiovascular health and coordination, while also being fun and social.
  Frequency: 150 minutes of moderate-intensity aerobic activity per week, or 75 minutes of vigorous-intensity aerobic activity.

Balance and Flexibility Exercises

As sarcopenia progresses, maintaining balance and flexibility becomes crucial to prevent falls and maintain independence. These practices improve flexibility, joint health, and balance, reducing the risk of falls and fractures. Enhanced mobility from these exercises allows older adults to stay active and perform strength training safely.

- **Yoga:** Helps improve balance, flexibility, and muscle tone, while also promoting relaxation. Poses like tree pose, warrior pose, and downward dog engage multiple muscle groups.
- **Tai Chi:** This low-impact exercise emphasizes controlled movements and balance, helping to improve coordination and reduce the risk of falls.
- **Pilates:** Focuses on core strength, flexibility, and alignment, making it an excellent choice for maintaining functional mobility and muscle control.
- **Balance Drills:** Simple activities such as standing on one leg, walking heel-to-toe, or using a stability ball can enhance balance and coordination.

Frequency: Two to three times a week for flexibility and balance exercises.

Modified High-Intensity Interval Training (HIIT)

Although high-intensity interval training (HIIT) workouts may seem challenging, a *modified HIIT* routine can be beneficial for many older adults, as recommended by their healthcare providers. It's important to be cautious and listen to your body, as some HIIT exercises like jumping jacks, burpees, and mountain climbers can be high-impact and potentially risky for older adults or those with joint or back issues. A safer approach is to adapt the HIIT exercises to *lower-impact versions* that still provide the benefits. For example, instead of high impact jumping jacks, you could do marching in place. Instead of burpees, you could do modified push-ups or squats without the jump. *The key is to focus on short bursts of moderate-to-high intensity exercise followed by rest periods.* This type of modified HIIT can help maintain muscle mass and improve cardiovascular health in older adults, as long as it's cleared by your physician and adjusted to your individual fitness level and health needs.

Additional Tips for Preventing Sarcopenia

- **Consistency:** Regular exercise is essential to prevent muscle deterioration. Even light exercises can help maintain muscle mass if done consistently. I advise my patients to start slow and that consistency is far better than perfection in this regard.
- **Progressive Overload:** Gradually increase the resistance or weight you lift to continuously challenge your muscles and stimulate growth.
- **Rest and Recovery:** Allow muscles to recover between strength training sessions to prevent injury and promote muscle repair.

Engaging in a well-rounded program that combines these forms of exercise can effectively prevent and treat sarcopenia, improving both strength and quality of life as you age. Exercise, especially resistance training, is essential not only for preventing sarcopenia but also for restoring muscle function and slowing the aging process.

―

As we conclude this chapter on exercise, it's clear that physical activity is an essential pillar of health, youthfulness, and longevity. By incorporating a variety of exercises—such as strength training, aerobic activities, and flexibility routines—into your daily life, you not only protect your body from the effects of aging but also support mental clarity, emotional well-being, and overall vitality. At its core it is a powerful tool to enhance both your lifespan and healthspan, allowing you to live a longer, healthier, and more vibrant life.

In the next chapter, we'll explore another crucial component of anti-aging and longevity: supplements and herbs. Just as exercise supports physical and mental health, certain supplements and natural remedies offer profound benefits for cellular health, immune function, and vitality. These scientifically backed compounds can be a key part of your wellness journey, helping you maintain youthfulness and health as you age. Let's dive into this wonderful world of nature's gifts to all of us and uncover how these can complement the benefits of exercise in your quest for lasting vitality.

CHAPTER 17

Supplements and Herbs: Secrets of Nature's Remedies

The time to repair the roof is when the sun is shining.
—John F. Kennedy, thirty-fifth president of the
United States (1917–1963)

Nature is pleased with simplicity. And
nature is no dummy.
—Sir Isaac Newton, The Principia: Mathematical
Principles of Natural Philosophy, British physicist and
mathematician (1643–1727)

Growing up in India, I was immersed in the use of supplements and herbs as part of the traditional Indian health system, *Ayurveda*. Now in my years of experience in regenerative and anti-aging medicine, I've seen firsthand the profound impact the right supplements and herbs can have on how we age. Whether you're aiming to increase your energy, protect brain function, or support overall cellular health, many scientifically backed natural compounds offer powerful tools to help you age gracefully and live with vitality.

Plants, herbs, and supplements are nature's gifts, designed to help us survive and thrive. As a matter of fact, the entire botanical ecosystem evolved alongside humanity and is significantly more ancient than we are. For thousands of years, plants have served as humanity's pharmacy, offering remedies that address a wide range of health concerns: from boosting the immune system and improving digestion to supporting anti-aging skin care.

When it comes to maintaining youthfulness and promoting longevity, supplements and herbs serve as a vital bridge between modern medicine and ancient wisdom. Through the years, I've come to appreciate the secrets of nature's remedies—many of which have been used for centuries in Ayurveda and other traditional healing practices such as traditional Chinese medicine, Mexico's *curanderismo*, Ancient CHamoru (or Chamorro) medicine, and Amazonian indigenous medicine. Today we have the advantage of not only understanding their time-tested uses but also uncovering the science behind why they work.

In this chapter, we will explore a few of the powerful, scientifically backed supplements and herbs that can help rejuvenate cells, support optimal brain and heart health, enhance energy levels, and ultimately extend both healthspan and lifespan. From the potent antioxidants found in resveratrol and curcumin to the adaptogenic properties of ashwagandha and ginseng, *these natural compounds have proven their ability to counteract the effects of aging at a cellular level.* Whether you're looking to reduce inflammation, protect against oxidative stress, boost cognitive function, or maintain vitality well into your later years, *the right combination of supplements and herbs can make a tangible difference in managing diseases and how you age.*

> For optimal results, the key is finding a perfect blend of herbs and supplements that is personalized for that particular person based on his or her medical history, biomarker tests, and medical needs.

While the following table does not encompass everything there is to know about herbs and supplements for optimal healthspan and longevity, it highlights some of the most proven and widely used options to help slow down aging and keep you feeling youthful.

Name	Action or Effect	Practical Tip
Fisetin The Senolytic Superhero (500 to 1,500 mg daily)	Fisetin clears senescent (zombie) cells, which accumulate with age and cause inflammation. Removing these cells promotes healthier aging and supports longevity.	Pair fisetin with quercetin for enhanced senolytic effects.
Pyrroloquinoline Quinone (PQQ) The Mitochondrial Mastermind (10 to 20 mg daily)	PQQ stimulates new mitochondrial production, boosting energy and cognitive function, making it essential for fighting fatigue and age-related decline.	Combine PQQ with CoQ10 for optimal mitochondrial support.
Nicotinamide Mononucleotide (NMN) Reversing Cellular Aging (250 to 1,000 mg daily)	NMN boosts NAD+ levels, improving cellular energy production and promoting DNA repair, crucial for aging healthily.	Take NMN with fisetin daily to enhance longevity and cellular health.
Glutathione The Master Antioxidant (250 to 1,000 mg daily)	Glutathione detoxifies cells and reduces oxidative stress. As levels decline with age, supplementing can protect against aging-related diseases.	Supplement this with resveratrol or NAC (N-Acetyl Cysteine) to boost antioxidant protection.
Pentadecylic Acid (C15:0) The Anti-Inflammatory Powerhouse (100 to 300 mg daily)	C15:0 reduces chronic inflammation, which is linked to aging and metabolic diseases.	Include this supplement to help lower inflammation. Take with turmeric for enhanced results.
Microdose Lithium Orotate Brain Health and Neuroprotection (0.3 to 1 mg daily)	Very low-dose lithium protects the brain, improving cognitive function and offering neuroprotection against aging-related decline.	Consult a physician before microdosing lithium for brain health.

Name	Action or Effect	Practical Tip
Triphala The Gut's Best Friend (500 to 1,000 mg daily)	Literally meaning "three fruits," this Ayurvedic blend of three herbs supports digestion, gut microbiome, and detoxification, all essential for aging well.	Take triphala daily in powder or capsule form. Add prebiotics and probiotics for extra boost.
Rhodiola A Natural Protector Against Senescent Cells (200 to 600 mg daily)	Rhodiola reduces stress and protects against cellular senescence, keeping cells youthful and supporting mental clarity.	Use rhodiola to reduce fatigue and promote athletic performance and recovery.
Tulsi (holy basil) The Stress Reliever (300 to 500 mg daily)	Tulsi reduces cortisol and helps balance the body's response to chronic stress, which accelerates aging.	Enjoy tulsi as a tea for stress relief.
Bacopa The Brain Booster (300 to 600 mg daily)	Bacopa enhances memory and cognitive function while preventing age-related cognitive decline.	Take bacopa daily to maintain sharpness and mental clarity.
Guduchi (*Tinospora cordifolia*) The Immune Enhancer (300 to 1,000 mg daily)	Guduchi boosts immunity, fights inflammation, and promotes longevity by strengthening the body's defenses.	Brew guduchi tea or take it in supplement form to boost your immune system.
Resveratrol The Longevity Molecule (1,500 to 2,000 mg daily)	Resveratrol activates longevity genes and mimics the effects of calorie restriction, supporting heart, brain health and anti-aging.	Take resveratrol supplements with Pterostilbene for added benefits.
Curcumin The Golden Spice of Life (500 to 2,000 mg daily)	Curcumin is a powerful anti-inflammatory and antioxidant, protecting against oxidative stress and supporting brain health.	Pair curcumin with black pepper to improve absorption. Watch for gastric upset.

Name	Action or Effect	Practical Tip
Coenzyme Q10 (CoQ10) The Cellular Energizer (100 to 200 mg daily)	CoQ10 boosts energy production and protects against cellular damage, which is crucial as natural levels decline with age.	CoQ10 is particularly important for those on statins, cholesterol lowering medicines.
Omega-3 Fatty Acids: Nourish the Heart and Mind (500 mg of combined EPA and DHA)	Omega-3s reduce inflammation, support heart health, and protect cognitive function, while also promoting skin elasticity. Important for anyone following a plant-based lifestyle.	Consider getting your omega-3 from flaxseeds and chia seeds.
Ashwagandha The Ancient Adaptogen (250 to 500 mg daily)	Ashwagandha reduces cortisol, boosts energy, and helps the body adapt to stress, improving overall resilience.	Take ashwagandha daily for energy and stress reduction. Great to combine with tulsi and guduchi.
Vitamin D_3 The Sunshine Vitamin (1,000 to 5,000 IU daily)	Vitamin D_3 is essential for bone health, immunity, and mood regulation, reducing the risk of chronic diseases. Linked to aging. I recommend this to all my patients, even if living in sunny areas such as Florida. More so if you are following a plant-based diet.	Supplement with vitamin D, especially in winter or if you have low sun exposure.
Melatonin Restoring Sleep and Beyond (3 – 10 mg daily)	Melatonin regulates sleep cycles and acts as an antioxidant, promoting restful sleep and healthy aging.	Use melatonin to regulate sleep and support recovery.

Name	Action or Effect	Practical Tip
Quercetin The Senolytic Agent (250 to 1,000 mg daily)	Quercetin reduces inflammation and oxidative stress and may help clear senescent cells, supporting healthy aging.	It complements other senolytic agents such as fisetin.
Pterostilbene Highly Bio-available Anti-oxidant (100 to 200 mg daily)	Found in blueberries and grapes, it offers several health benefits, including reducing oxidative stress, preventing certain cancers, supporting neurological and heart health, fighting inflammation, boosting immunity, combating infections, and aiding diabetes management.	It complements other antioxidant agents such as resveratrol.

Some Resources for Additional Information

As most of you already know, there is an abundance of information available on herbs and supplements online, and those interested in exploring herbal remedies can start with reputable sources. Here are some of the websites for you to learn authentic information on herbs and supplements for health and longevity:

- **National Center for Complementary and Integrative Health:** The NCCIH provides reliable information on various herbs and supplements, including research summaries and safety information. Website: https://www.nccih.nih.gov/.
- **NIH Office of Dietary Supplements:** The ODS detailed fact sheets on various supplements. Website: https://ods.od.nih.gov/.

- **American Botanical Council:** Offers a wealth of information on herbal medicine and research. Website: https://abc.herbalgram.org/.
- **WebMD:** Provides trustworthy health information, including articles on herbs, supplements, and their benefits. Website: https://www.webmd.com/.
- **Mayo Clinic:** Provides reliable health information and research on herbs and supplements. Website: https://www.mayoclinic.org/drugs-supplements.
- **Johns Hopkins Medicine:** Provides comprehensive information on dietary supplements and their health benefits. Website: https://www.hopkinsmedicine.org/health/wellness-and-prevention/dietary-supplements.
- **Stanford University School of Medicine:** offers research and articles on various supplements and their effects. Website: https://longevity.stanford.edu/lifestyle/2024/03/11/supplements-for-healthy-aging/.
- **Memorial Sloan Kettering Cancer Center:** Designated a comprehensive cancer center by the National Cancer Institute, MSKCC provides first-rate research on most of the commonly used supplements and herbs. Website: https://www.mskcc.org/cancer-care/diagnosis-treatment/symptom-management/integrative-medicine/herbs/search.

Before starting any new supplement, I recommend *consulting with a healthcare provider such as an herbalist or naturalist* to ensure that your regimen is aligned with your unique health and longevity goals. By incorporating these supplements and herbs as part of your holistic longevity protocol, as I use in VitalLife, you can enhance cellular repair, boost brain function, strengthen immune resilience, and better manage stress. I've witnessed many patients experience significant benefits from this combined approach, which unites the latest scientific findings with time-honored remedies.

As we've discussed, supplements and herbs provide powerful support for physical health and promote vitality. But true longevity also depends on nourishing the mind and emotions. Our mental and emotional health plays a critical role in how we live daily and age, influencing everything from how we manage stress to how resilient we are in the face of life's challenges. In the next chapter, we'll explore mindfulness as well as the role of sleep in health and longevity. Let's dive into how to bring calm, clarity, and emotional resilience, setting the foundation for a stress-free, peaceful lifestyle.

CHAPTER 18

The Power of Mindfulness and Restful Sleep: A Stress-Free, Energetic Life

You only have power over your mind—not outside events. Realize this, and you will find strength.
—Marcus Aurelius, Roman emperor and Stoic philosopher (AD 121–80)

We don't see things as they are, we see them as we are.
— Anaïs Nin, French-born American writer (1903–1977)

A senior monk and a junior monk were traveling together when they came upon a river with a strong current. As they prepared to cross, they noticed a young, beautiful woman struggling at the riverbank, clearly hesitant about how to make it across. She turned to them and asked for their help. The monks exchanged a glance, knowing they had taken vows not to touch a woman. Without a word, the senior monk stepped forward, lifted the woman onto his shoulders, and carried her across the river. Once they reached the other side, he gently set her down, nodded politely, and continued on his journey. The younger monk was stunned. He walked alongside his companion in complete silence, the events replaying in his mind. An hour passed, then another, and yet another.

Finally, unable to hold back any longer, the younger monk blurted out, "As monks, we've taken vows not to touch a woman. How could you carry her on your shoulders?" The older monk paused, turned to him, and said with a calm, knowing smile, "Brother, I set her down on the other side of the river long time ago. Why are you still carrying her?"

America, the Land of Opportunity

America is a place where dreams are pursued and often realized, where the promise of a better life draws people, including myself, from around the world. This promise is evident in its creativity, innovation, and ability to empower individuals to achieve what once seemed impossible. America is celebrated as the land of opportunity—opportunity to become successful, where money, power, and fame are within reach for anyone willing to pursue them. We in America are laser focused on the relentless pursuit of achieving success, sometimes by all means possible and at any cost. And soon life itself becomes nothing else but an unending chase for success. I have seen it, I have been there.

While this pursuit may deliver comfort, luxury, and material possessions, it is a double-edged sword. As darkness follows light, it comes glued with unyielding anxiety, crushing stress, and an endless rush through life. Like a hamster on a wheel, we seem to be always struggling and rushing to reach nowhere. In America we have so many beautiful gardens, but most of us have no time, intention, or patience to slow down and really enjoy these gardens, no time to simply "stop and smell the roses." I have seen it, I have been there.

Astonishingly, though they make up just 4.2 percent of the world's population, Americans devour a colossal share of pills for anxiety, for depression, for sleep, for pain. Layer this with the ruthless tide of illicit drugs and addictions, and what emerges is not merely an ultra-wealthy, most powerful nation on the surface but, at its hollow core, a restless soul weeping in the dark—yearning for love, grasping for connection, yet sinking deeper into its own loneliness. This too I have seen, I have been there.

> As I grow older, I've come to realize how much time I've wasted in this ceaseless, fruitless pursuit of success. For many of us, this relentless chase becomes the very obstacle to truly knowing and living life.
> *You see, in this way, we are the sole jailers of our own "life."*

In this constant pursuit to acquire money, power, success, and fame, the challenge lies in recognizing the *value of "enough"* and *embracing a life that prioritizes* family over a fattening wallet, meaning over materialism, connection over consumption, and well-being over wealth. I have no answer to America's hallucination of a *"constant rush to instant success"* psyche, except to quote someone who knew a thing or two: Albert Einstein once wisely said, "A calm and modest life brings more happiness than the pursuit of success combined with constant restlessness."

Having practiced mindfulness since early childhood, I can tell you this with deep conviction: *a mindfulness lifestyle can help us rediscover calm, peace, and joy*—without relying on any drugs. My own journey with mindfulness began as early as I can remember, around the age of five or six, when I was first introduced to the practices of meditation and yoga. While growing up in India, these activities were not considered extraordinary; they were simply an integral part of daily life. Mindfulness wasn't something we sought out intentionally; it was simply a way of living. Meditation and yoga were as essential to our routine as the food we ate or the air we breathed. *They were woven into the fabric of our culture*, shaping how we connected with ourselves, our families, and the world around us. These practices nurtured mental clarity, emotional balance, and a deep sense of peace from an early age—a foundation that has guided me throughout my life and career.

These mindfulness techniques, which are now cornerstones in modern wellness, were simply part of life for us in India. Just as we added turmeric, cumin, coriander, and ginger to our curry to promote healing and wellness, we also turned to mindfulness practices to maintain balance and harmony of mind, body, and soul. The same way turmeric supported our physical health, meditation and yoga nurtured our emotional and mental well-being, helping us manage stress, sharpen our focus, and cultivate a lasting sense of calm. Looking back, I can see how these early lessons in mindfulness laid the foundation for the vitality I experience today—and how they continue to shape my approach to health as a physician.

A Few Fundamentals to Consider Before Starting a Mindfulness Practice

From my own experience practicing mindfulness since childhood, I can tell you that no matter what technique you choose to adopt—whether it's meditation, yoga, or simple breath awareness—*there are a few fundamentals that apply to all*. I find that the best results from any mindfulness technique come when we *approach it with an open heart and a willingness to let go*. Let go of the rush, the need for control, and the endless demands that pull us in a hundred directions. Let go of the guilts, grudges, and regrets of the past. The story at the beginning of this chapter was shared with me by a learned Zen master in Toronto, Canada, several years ago. He also told me—"*Let go or be dragged.*" I've always been drawn to its simplicity and the profound calm it brings—an ability to find peace by letting go of what I cannot control.

This "letting go" mirrors the core of Stoic philosophy, where the *dichotomy of control teaches us to focus on what we can influence—our thoughts, actions, and reactions—while releasing the grip on external events and others' behavior that we have no control over*. It's a practice that fosters serenity amidst life's chaos. Mindfulness, for me, is a powerful tool to embrace this philosophy and cultivate a steady, peaceful state of mind.

> Without even realizing it, we spend much of our waking hours consumed by grudges, guilt, and regrets about the past or worrying about and planning for the future. Mindfulness invites you to experience the transformational "power of the present."

True mindfulness thrives in simplicity: pause for just a few minutes throughout the day, breathe deeply, and truly notice the world around you. Stop and smell the roses—literally. Feel the sun on your face, the rhythm of your breath, or the joy in a small act of kindness. *Giving*, whether it's your time, a smile, or an act of service, creates space for gratitude and connection, enriching your practice. It's not about perfection or long hours of meditation; *it's about reconnecting with the ordinary and allowing yourself to slow down enough to truly experience it.*

I often tell my patients that *mindfulness isn't just about quieting the mind; it's about cultivating a deeper connection with oneself*. Regular mindfulness practice reduces stress, anxiety, and depression while promoting a positive outlook on life. By *weaving mindfulness into your daily routine*, you give yourself the tools to live with clarity, balance, and inner peace, helping you navigate life's challenges with greater ease.

Simple things like *cultivating a lifestyle that invites calmness* into our daily routine are essential. And, experiencing the "power of the present"—this includes being mindful of the food we consume, being attentive in everything we do at home or work, and being fully present when spending precious time with our loved ones. *Embracing gratitude* is another cornerstone—taking moments each day to appreciate what we already have, instead of just focusing on all that more we need and desire. Appreciating the blessings, both big and small, can always shift my perspective and open my heart.

What Zen masters, monks, sadhus, and gurus have understood for centuries is now being validated by modern science. Practicing mindfulness cultivates a profound sense of presence and calm, which can transform the way we navigate the stresses of daily life. Over the years of practicing medicine, I have seen that *patients who incorporate mindfulness report feeling more grounded, resilient, calmer, and better equipped to handle life's demands*. It is interesting that many times family members, friends, and coworkers of the patient notice these benefits even before patient does.

I've found mindfulness to be one of the most powerful tools for enhancing not only emotional but also physical health. Science confirms these experiences—mindfulness has been shown to lower blood pressure, reduce inflammation, and strengthen immune function, all of which are critical for longevity and overall well-being. When we're fully present, the body can heal and function more optimally, creating a foundation for a vibrant and healthy life.

Let me share another Zen story with you:

Two young fish swam upstream, struggling against the current, when an older fish drifted by, nodding casually. "Well, boys, the water is so calm today!" he said. The young fish exchanged confused glances before one finally asked, *"What's 'water'?"*

I find this simple story profoundly meaningful, a reminder of *how easily we take the essentials for granted.* Just like fish, completely immersed in water yet unaware of its presence, we too often fail to recognize the fundamental elements that sustain and shape our very existence. In the hustle of daily life—caught up in deadlines, responsibilities, and the relentless pursuit of survival and success—we forget to truly live. We overlook the beauty around us, the breath we take, the relationships that anchor us, and the small joys that make life extraordinary. We are simply too rushed to see the true abundance around us, the very fabric of our being.

> We consistently overlook the beauty and abundance around us. In the hustle of daily life—caught up in deadlines, responsibilities, and the relentless pursuit of survival and success—we forget to truly live.

I wholeheartedly believe that *life isn't just about success and surviving; it's about awakening to the richness of our daily existence and savoring what's right in front of us.* This awareness, though simple, can transform how we approach each day, reconnecting us to what truly matters.

One other important feature to remember: *mindfulness isn't about chasing brief moments of calm*; it's a lifestyle that is proven for reducing stress, improving mental clarity, and enhancing emotional balance. Research consistently shows that mindfulness reduces anxiety, improves emotional regulation, and lowers the risk of depression, making it an essential tool for improving health and longevity.

Remember, mindfulness is not about achieving a specific state or outcome; it's about being present, fully and authentically. By integrating these fundamentals into your chosen technique, you create a solid foundation that supports deeper awareness and a more profound connection with yourself. The journey is uniquely yours, but these guiding principles can help illuminate the path toward greater peace and understanding.

Let's now explore some of the most effective and scientifically proven mindfulness techniques and how they can be seamlessly integrated into everyday life for optimal well-being.

A Few Key Techniques for Mindfulness

A relaxed state of mind and body is crucial for any mindfulness practice. Before you begin, allow yourself to settle into a comfortable position, letting go of any physical tension or mental clutter. Approach your practice as a *gentle observer*, being a *"witness"* to your thoughts and sensations *without any judgment*. This means acknowledging whatever arises—be it calmness, restlessness, joy, or discomfort—with acceptance and compassion.

> Remember, mindfulness is not about achieving a specific state or outcome. It is about being present, fully and authentically. Approach your practice as a gentle observer, being a nonjudgmental witness.

I encourage focusing on simple, foundational techniques that are easily available and scientifically validated. There's no shortage of apps, websites, and techniques available to support mindfulness practices. Let's discuss some of the most popular ones now:

Meditation Techniques: Cultivating Present Moment Awareness

Meditation is one of the most well-known mindfulness practices, and it's supported by decades of research. Regular meditation has been shown to reduce stress, lower blood pressure, improve attention, and even slow the aging of the brain. Techniques like *focused attention meditation, mantra meditation, and mindfulness meditation* train the mind to focus on the present moment, bringing a deep sense of calm and mental clarity. Studies have found that consistent meditation can change brain structure, increasing the density of gray matter in regions associated with memory, empathy, and emotional regulation.

Practical Tip: Start with just five to ten minutes of meditation practice once or twice a day, focusing on your breath or using a simple mantra like "om," or "Christ," or "so hum," to center your mind.

Yoga: The Mind-Body Connection

The Sanskrit word for *yoga* is *yuj*, which means "to unite." Yoga is more than just a physical exercise—it is a practice that unites body, thoughts, attention, and breath. An enormous amount of clinical studies over the past several decades have shown what sages in India have known for thousands of years: that yoga reduces stress, cultivates calm, improves flexibility, enhances mental focus, and even boosts immune function. It integrates mindfulness into physical movement, promoting awareness of the body and its sensations. Medical research confirms that yoga can lower cortisol levels, the hormone linked to stress, and improve emotional balance by enhancing brain plasticity.

Practical Tip: Incorporate yoga into your weekly routine, even if it's just a few minutes of stretching and mindful breathing each day.

Deep Breathing Exercises: Calm at Your Fingertips

One of the simplest yet most powerful mindfulness techniques is deep breathing. Breathing exercises, such as *diaphragmatic breathing* (taking slow, deep breaths using your diaphragm) and *4-7-8 breathing* (inhaling for 4 seconds, holding the breath for 7 seconds, and exhaling for 8 seconds), are scientifically proven to activate the parasympathetic nervous system and Vagus nerve, promoting relaxation and lowering stress levels. By focusing on slow, controlled breaths, you can lower your heart rate and reduce anxiety almost instantly. These exercises are particularly beneficial for lowering blood pressure, improving lung function, and enhancing mental clarity.

Practical Tip: Practice deep breathing for five to ten minutes multiple times a day, particularly during stressful moments, to promote immediate calm and focus.

Body Scan: Awareness of the Body and Its Sensations

Derived from one aspect of Buddhist Vipassana meditation, the body scan is a mindfulness technique that involves mentally *scanning* the body from head to toe, paying attention to physical sensations without judgment. This practice encourages deep relaxation, reduces muscle tension, and heightens awareness of the mind-body connection. Studies show that body scanning can improve sleep quality, reduce chronic pain, and increase overall well-being by promoting a state of deep relaxation and body awareness.

Practical Tip: Try a ten-minute body scan before bed or after a stressful day to promote relaxation and improve sleep quality.

Living in the Present Moment

As we discussed earlier, most of us spend the majority of our time thinking about the guilt and regrets of the past and worrying or planning about the future. By staying present, we can become more attuned to our mental and emotional state, allowing us to respond to stressors with greater calm and clarity. This simple technique of "focusing on the present" has been linked to improved cognitive function and emotional resilience, which are crucial for aging gracefully as well.

Practical Tip: This technique can be easily incorporated throughout the day, whether during a walk, while eating, or simply during daily tasks by paying full attention to the present moment.

Technological Tools in Mindfulness: Apps to Keep You on Track

With advances in technology, mindfulness has become more accessible than ever. Apps like *Calm, Headspace, and Smiling Mind* offer guided meditations, breathing exercises, and body scan sessions that make it easy to incorporate mindfulness into a busy day. These apps may require subscriptions and provide structured programs that fit into any schedule, allowing you to practice mindfulness on the go. From my experience, I've seen that mindfulness apps are *particularly effective for beginners or those looking to build a consistent practice.* Multiple studies have shown that these apps can help reduce anxiety, improve sleep quality, and promote emotional well-being, making them valuable tools for anyone wanting to enhance their mental and emotional health.

In addition to these apps I mentioned, there are many other free online resources on mindfulness techniques, including guided meditation, yoga, deep breathing, body scans, and modern approaches to mindfulness. These tools make it easier to explore various techniques, so you can find the ones that resonate best with your goals for relaxation, focus, or stress management. I am listing a few below to learn more about mindfulness and yoga. These resources offer a variety of tools and techniques to support mindfulness practice, making it easy for you to explore and implement these methods into your life. These sites can give you accessible, practical information on mindfulness techniques to support your journey toward better mental and emotional health.

Mindful.org—Mindfulness Practices URL: https://www.mindful.org	Mindful.org offers a wide range of articles, guides, and resources on mindfulness practices such as meditation, deep breathing, and body scan techniques. It also includes practical tips for incorporating mindfulness into daily life.
Yoga Journal—Mindfulness and Yoga Practices https://www.yogajournal.com	Yoga Journal is a comprehensive resource for all things yoga, with specific sections dedicated to mindfulness practices like meditation and deep breathing.
The Chopra Center—Meditation and Mindfulness https://chopra.com/articles/meditation	The Chopra Center offers detailed guides on various mindfulness techniques, including meditation, breathing exercises, and yoga. They emphasize the mind-body connection and provide tools for integrating mindfulness into daily routines.
The American Institute of Stress—Relaxation and Mindfulness Techniques https://www.stress.org	The American Institute of Stress offers scientifically supported mindfulness techniques like meditation and deep breathing to reduce stress and improve emotional well-being.
UCLA Health's Mindfulness Education Center https://www.ucla-health.org/uclamindful	This center is advancing mindfulness education worldwide. It provides evidence-based mindfulness programs that empower people to manage stress, enhance health, and cultivate inner peace.

A Special Note on the Epidemic of Loneliness in America

In 2023 a surgeon general's advisory raised an alarm about the devastating impact of the epidemic of loneliness and isolation in United States. It is a growing crisis in the United States, with surveys revealing that *nearly one in three adults* often feels lonely. This isn't just an emotional concern—it's a significant public health issue. Research shows that chronic loneliness is as detrimental to health as smoking fifteen cigarettes a day, contributing to heart disease, stroke, depression, and even premature death. It weakens the immune system, increases inflammation, leads to chronic stress and anxiety, and accelerates cognitive decline, making it a silent but powerful factor in poor health and aging.

> Research shows that chronic loneliness is as detrimental to health as smoking fifteen cigarettes a day, contributing to heart disease, stroke, depression, and even premature death.

It's important to distinguish between living alone and feeling lonely. Many people, including myself, cherish their independence and find joy in solitude. Living alone doesn't have to mean loneliness. The key lies in maintaining meaningful social connections and a sense of purpose, which are vital for mental and physical well-being.

Simple steps can make a profound difference—have meaningful social connections, reach out to friends or family, join community groups or clubs, or volunteer for a cause you care about. Practicing gratitude, adopting a pet, or engaging in shared activities like group exercise or hobby classes can also help build connections and combat the epidemic of loneliness. It's about creating a life rich in relationships and experiences, ensuring that no one feels invisible or forgotten in a fast-paced, often isolating world.

I would like to add here the amazing benefits of pet ownership, especially as it relates to loneliness. As loneliness emerges as a pressing public health challenge, pet ownership offers a meaningful way to combat its effects. Pets provide steadfast companionship, filling emotional gaps and creating a sense of connection that is often lost in times of isolation. Research from esteemed institutions such as Harvard and Johns Hopkins highlights the science behind these benefits, pointing to the release of oxytocin—the "love hormone"—during positive interactions with pets. This hormone, which fosters social bonding and emotional warmth, is triggered through simple acts like petting a dog or playing with a cat. It not only promotes relaxation but also reduces stress indicators like high blood pressure and heart rate, supporting overall well-being.

Beyond these physiological effects, pets play a pivotal role in alleviating the emotional and psychological burdens of loneliness. They offer unwavering affection and companionship, while also bringing a sense of purpose and structure to daily life through caregiving routines. Moreover, pets serve as social bridges, helping their owners connect with others in shared spaces, such as dog parks, or through participation in pet-focused communities. By addressing both the emotional and social aspects of loneliness, pets become invaluable allies—not just in managing isolation, but in fostering joy and reconnection. For pet owners, the bond forged with their furry friends is truly life-enhancing.

Sound, Restful Sleep: Sleep Hygiene

In all my years of practice, I've seen how restful, sound sleep is one of the most important—and often underestimated—factors for longevity, energy, and optimal health. I've seen countless patients struggling with low energy, mood swings, and poor cognitive function, unaware that the quality of their sleep was often at the root of these issues. Without the right amount of restorative sleep, your body simply can't perform at its best—it's like trying to power through the day on a depleted battery. I'll admit, if I don't get at least six hours of deep, uninterrupted sleep, you definitely don't want to be around me the next day.

Sleep is not just about recharging for the next day—*it's the time your body needs to heal, regenerate, and prepare for the challenges ahead.* During deep sleep, the body enters full repair mode. It's when your hormones are balanced, your immune system is strengthened, and your cells have the chance to regenerate. This is the time when growth hormone surges, helping to repair tissues, build muscle, and even manage metabolism. If you're not sleeping well, all of these critical functions are disrupted. Over time, poor sleep can lead to serious issues like insulin resistance, weight gain, and an increased risk of chronic diseases like diabetes or heart disease. But when you get the restorative sleep your body craves, you wake up recharged, with improved energy, focus, and resilience to handle stress.

> During deep sleep, the body enters full repair mode. It's when your hormones are balanced, your immune system is strengthened, and the cells in your body repair and regenerate.

Quality sleep benefits not only physical health but mental and emotional well-being, too. When you're well rested, your brain has had time to process information, regulate emotions, and consolidate memories. That's why I emphasize to my patients that sleep is a crucial part of maintaining sharp cognitive function and mental clarity. Whether it's performing at work, staying focused during the day, or even building emotional resilience, sleep plays a foundational role. And let's not forget: consistent, deep sleep has been shown to protect against cognitive decline and diseases like Alzheimer's.

The key, however, isn't just about clocking in more hours—it's about the quality of your sleep. Sound, quality sleep is one of the most powerful tools we have for supporting longevity, youthfulness, and peak performance in every area of life. And once you make it a priority, you'll be amazed at how it transforms your daily experience. I always emphasize the importance of *creating a sleep routine, optimizing your sleep environment, managing stress, and also considering diet, supplements, and herbs for sound sleep.* By prioritizing these elements, you give your body the best chance to recover and thrive.

- **Sleep Routine:** Achieving restful, sound sleep is more than just going to bed every night—it's about creating an environment and routine that allows your body and mind to truly unwind and recover. The first step I recommend is creating a consistent sleep routine. Going to bed and waking up at the same time every day helps to regulate your body's internal clock, or circadian rhythm. When your body knows what to expect, it's easier to fall asleep, stay asleep, and wake up feeling refreshed. Consistency, even on weekends, makes a big difference in how your body adapts to a regular sleep pattern.
- **Sleep Environment:** The sleeping environment is just as important. Your bedroom should be a sanctuary for rest—quiet, dark, and cool. These small adjustments have a huge impact on the quality of your sleep. I often tell patients to avoid all digital screens (phones, tablets, or TVs) at least an hour before bed. The blue light emitted by screens tricks your brain into thinking it's still daytime, which can interfere with the production of melatonin, the hormone that signals your body that it's time to sleep. Instead, I encourage incorporating relaxing bedtime rituals like reading a book, practicing deep breathing, or even a light stretching routine to help wind down.
- **Stress Management:** Another key element is stress management. Throughout the day, many of us carry around a significant amount of stress that we don't release,

and this can carry over into the night, making it harder to fall asleep or stay asleep. Engaging in practices like mindfulness, as we discussed above, or journaling before bed can help quiet the mind and calm the nervous system. When your mind is relaxed, your body follows, allowing you to drift into a more peaceful, restorative sleep.

- **Herbs and Supplements:** In addition to these habits, certain herbs and supplements can be extremely beneficial in promoting restful sleep. For example, *melatonin* supplements are often used to help regulate sleep cycles, especially for those who may struggle with falling asleep or staying asleep. *Chamomile*, known for its calming effects, can also be a wonderful addition to your evening routine. Drinking chamomile tea before bed can help soothe the nervous system, preparing your body for a deeper, more restful sleep. Other herbs like *valerian root* and *passionflower* have also been shown to support relaxation and improve sleep quality. Incorporating these natural aids can be an excellent way to gently support your body's natural sleep processes.
- **Diet:** As with so many other things, diet also plays a role in sleep quality. What you eat and drink, especially in the evening, can either support or hinder restful sleep. I often recommend avoiding caffeine or heavy meals close to bedtime, as both can disrupt your ability to fall asleep. Instead, a light snack rich in tryptophan—like almonds, cashews, or other nuts—can help promote better sleep by boosting melatonin levels. Staying hydrated throughout the day is essential too but cutting off fluids an hour or two before bed can prevent those middle-of-the-night trips to the bathroom.

By incorporating these proven mindfulness and restful sleep strategies into your daily life, you can not only manage stress and improve emotional health but also support your overall physical well-being. Whether through traditional practices like yoga and meditation or using modern tools like apps, the *key is consistency*. From my own experience growing up with these practices and seeing their scientifically proven benefits, I am convinced that incorporating mindfulness into daily life can profoundly improve health and longevity.

As we move forward in this journey, it's important to reflect on how these lifestyle modification tools we've discussed—ranging from plant-based diet and supplements to mindfulness—can work together to optimize overall well-being. These strategies form the core of a holistic approach to living longer, healthier, and more vibrantly. In the final section of this book, we'll draw conclusions about this journey and how you can implement these practices to unlock your body's full potential and live a life of lasting vitality.

PART 5
CONCLUSION: A JOURNEY OF REJUVENATION

CHAPTER 19

Your 6-Step Action Plan for Youthfulness and Longevity

All the world is full of suffering. It is also full of overcoming.
—*Helen Keller, American blind and deaf writer and humanitarian (1880–1968)*

It's not what happens to you, but how you react to it that matters.
—*Epictetus, Greek Stoic philosopher (ca. AD 55–135)*

Now that we've explored all aspects of VitalLife program, you understand the scientific foundation of the program and the individual components that work together to deliver the best possible results. You've gained a comprehensive understanding of its features—from biomarker testing and regenerative treatments to addressing the Aging Triad and implementing lifestyle modifications—all designed to optimize health, reverse disease, and extend your healthspan.

Just like for so many others over these past many years, I'm confident that VitalLife will be a turning point for anyone seeking to rejuvenate their vitality and well-being for years to come. One patient, a former professional athlete in his forties, regained the energy and strength of his twenties through regenerative therapies, peptide optimization, and an anti-inflammatory regimen. Another, a high-profile CEO in his sixties, reversed years of burnout and cognitive decline by addressing insulin resistance and optimizing his brain health. These are not isolated cases—they're proof that when you target the root causes of aging with a comprehensive, personalized approach, a real lasting transformation is possible. It's the kind of transformation I envision for you as well.

I feel a word of caution is necessary here. It amazes me how dedicated people are to providing excellent care for their pets, yet often neglect the same level of care for themselves. While there are legitimate telemedicine e-clinics run by experienced physicians, I must strongly warn you to avoid many of the online platforms that focus on anti-aging, hormones, and youthfulness but operate solely as business ventures. These platforms often gain popularity by offering cheaper alternatives, but I've witnessed countless horror stories of people experiencing serious side effects from products like rapamycin, testosterone, or other anti-aging drugs purchased from these sources.

Your 6-Step Action Plan to Reverse Biological Age and Optimize Healthspan

We discussed the six pillars of this program in chapter 4. Each of these six pillars is carefully designed to work together, thus building a foundation for your lasting health. *These pillars form the 6-step action plan for you to design your own youthfulness and longevity program.*

Design Your Own Multifaceted Approach for Maximum Impact

Nothing compares to the personalized, compassionate care of an experienced physician who understands your unique needs and prioritizes your health and wellness—your most valuable asset. To achieve long-term success safely, it's essential to trust your health to a qualified professional. The best approach is to find an experienced physician in your area who specializes in regenerative and anti-aging medicine to act as your guide and consultant in this important journey. Armed with the knowledge of VitalLife, now you are ready to craft your own health plan that is:

- **Data-Driven:** testing biomarkers and retesting at regular intervals.
- **Comprehensive and Multifaceted:** Combining, as appropriate, targeted elements from all or many of the six steps discussed below.
- **Personalized:** Based on your tests, biology, and goals.
- **Updated Periodically:** Based on clinical response and biomarkers.

One more important factor to keep in mind. As we discussed in detail in chapter 6, the processes of aging and age-related diseases begin as early as our teenage years. *In essence, these are diseases of childhood showing up in later years.* Therefore, starting this program at a younger age, with a focus on prevention, requires significantly less effort compared to attempting to reverse a disease and regaining energy and vitality later in life.

> The processes of aging and age-related diseases—such as heart disease, stroke, diabetes, and Alzheimer's—begin as early as our teenage years, influenced by genetics, lifestyle, and environmental factors. In essence, these are diseases of childhood showing up in later years.

A few guidelines about how to implement this program for your health based on your age and disease, if any.

For People Under Forty with No Disease: When the focus is on prevention of diseases, especially for those under forty, two essential components are regular biomarker testing (step 1) and lifestyle modifications (step 6). These two steps form the foundation of disease prevention and optimal health during the early stages of life.

For People Under Forty with a Disease: If you have been diagnosed with a disease at a younger age, additional steps in the program may play a pivotal role. For instance, psychedelics have shown transformative potential for patients with PTSD, traumatic brain injuries, and treatment-resistant depression. Similarly, anti-inflammatory protocols are essential for managing autoimmune conditions such as long COVID, fibromyalgia, chronic fatigue syndrome, and lupus. For those dealing with resistant obesity or prediabetes, prioritizing the treatment of mitochondrial dysfunction and insulin resistance is crucial for achieving meaningful progress.

For People over Forty (Whether or Not You Have Been Diagnosed with a Disease): As you begin to experience the effects of aging, usually around the age of forty, such as low energy, reduced strength, or brain fog—or if you've been diagnosed with conditions like diabetes, heart disease, stroke, any auto-immune disease, or Alzheimer's, your treatment plan needs to be more aggressive. By this stage, the disease processes have often been progressing for years, if not decades. In these cases, I recommend utilizing at least few strategies from ALL six steps of the VitalLife program to achieve the best possible results.

—

Let me now summarize these six steps, which are important for your own health and longevity program.

1. Start with Biomarker Tests for a Personalized Plan

First decide your goals and reasons to achieve your goals. As we discussed, your own program must be fundamentally personalized, so start your own health plan based on objective data from biomarker testing and biological age assessments. I find that *you cannot change what you cannot measure.* As we discussed in chapter 7, these tests provide insights into how your body is functioning beneath the surface, so consider the biomarkers to find out whether your cells are fighting toxins in your body, your hormones are imbalanced, your inflammation levels are high, or your insulin sensitivity needs improvement. And don't forget the *DNA methylation biological age tests* such as Elysium and TruAge. *For heart concerns*, it is better to also check hs-CRP, ApoB, and LipoA instead of only relying on a traditional lipid profile. For assessing *metabolic health*, it is important to evaluate fasting glucose, insulin levels, c-peptide levels, HbA1c, HOMA-IR, and leptin levels. *Chronic inflammation markers* such as hs-CRP, ESR, complements, and ferritin levels are also helpful. When suspecting any *autoimmune diseases*, it is important to check specific biomarkers, including anti-ds DNA, rheumatoid factor, and antinuclear antibody.

Over the years, I have found using new MedTech devices to be quite helpful, especially Libre 3 continuous glucose monitor for insulin resistance (even in patients who don't have diabetes or obesity), Oura for quality of sleep, KardiaMobile for irregular heart rhythm (common in elderly patients and usually asymptomatic), and sleep apnea monitors.

Armed with this data, you can craft a treatment plan that is tailored to your unique biology and goals, ensuring that you get the exact care you need to achieve rejuvenation and long-term health. It is important to have your physician *repeat the biomarker tests on a regular basis* so that he or she can assess your progress, ensure the safety of the products used, and make modifications as needed for a best possible outcome.

2. Regenerative Modalities for Cellular Regeneration

Review the various regenerative treatments discussed in great detail in chapters 8 and 9. The key to optimal results is utilizing the synergy between various regenerative modalities, each playing a crucial role in restoring youthfulness and vitality. Based on your medical history, goals, and biomarker tests, *several of these cutting-edge regenerative therapies*, including *stem cells and exosomes*, can be great options for you and you should consider these by consulting an experienced physician in this field.

I have found often a *plan that combines several of these modalities* can be very helpful—such as integrating stem cell and exosome treatments, senolytic agents, IV infusions of NAD+, hyperbaric oxygen, and even plasma exchanges. And, as in VitalLife, also integrating these with metabolic, anti-inflammation, hormone balancing, and lifestyle modifications provides the best possible results for you. When these therapies are combined, they can have powerful effects to restore your health and to reverse age-related damage and diseases. In doing so, we not only slow the aging process but reverse some of the damage that has already been done. Patients who have undergone regenerative treatments with this integrated anti-aging approach often report feeling younger, with less pain, more energy, better cognition, and a greater sense of vitality.

Psychedelics can be a promising option if you have certain illnesses such as treatment-resistant depression, prolonged grief, chronic pain, incurable cancer, PTSD, or traumatic brain injury. If you have any of these concerns, discuss with a qualified physician to see if psychedelics are a safe and effective treatment for you. Compounds such as psilocybin and ketamine should be considered only as part of the overall treatment plan. For *psilocybin*, you can contact a few research institutions in the United States, such as NYU Langone, Johns Hopkins, and the University of California, San Francisco (UCSF). You can search the NIH's ClinicalTrials.gov website to find ongoing patient trials. Several centers in Oregon and Colorado are actively using psilocybin to help people with multiple health conditions. For those who can afford it, several retreats in Costa Rica and Europe offer psilocybin or magic mushroom journeys. Make sure to check the legal status of psilocybin or other psychedelic treatments in the country you plan to visit.

For *ketamine* treatment for the conditions listed above, there are several centers around the country as well as few authentic online platforms (such as *Mindbloom.com* and *Joyous.team*). It is a good idea to first check the source of the pharmacy they use and their licensing status through state medical board websites. With your physician, you can consider an *intermittent dosing protocol*, where we use therapeutic doses to actively manage various conditions by giving a dose two to three times a week for a limited time. Or alternatively use newer approach of daily *microdosing* or *very-low-dose (VLD) therapy*.

3. Hormone and Peptide Optimization

One of the key pillars of this program we discussed extensively is hormone and peptide optimization. Guided by blood and saliva tests, hormone and peptide optimization can help symptoms like fatigue, decrease in muscle mass and strength, brain fog, weight gain, and a decline in libido and sexual health. It is important to find a physician who does not simply replace testosterone injections or female bioidentical hormone creams to fix some blood tests but specializes in *comprehensive and personalized hormone and peptide optimization protocols* to restore hormone levels to their optimal balance. These products are important not just for turning back the clock but also to restore your body's internal environment to one that supports optimal cellular function.

It is important not to forget gonadorelin, anastrozole, or clomiphene with any testosterone treatment for men. Oxytocin, sermorelin, and low-dose testosterone for women have emerged as key components of this optimization protocol. *Equally important is incorporating support for the metabolic system, gut health, and cellular mitochondrial function.* These are foundational elements that determine how efficiently your body utilizes the hormones and peptides introduced during therapy. By addressing these interconnected systems, you set the foundation for not just hormonal balance but also long-term outcomes.

Remember, regular testing is essential to ensure the effectiveness and safety of hormone optimization as part of comprehensive medical care.

4. Controlling the Aging Triad of Mitochondrial Dysfunction, Metabolic Insulin Resistance, and Chronic Inflammation

We discussed in chapters 12 and 13 how to address these key components of the Aging Triad, which is the root cause of aging and chronic diseases.

By following a whole-food, plant-based diet with no processed foods, and reducing your fried foods and refined sugar, you can improve insulin sensitivity and allow your body to burn fat more efficiently as well as decrease inflammation. Strategies to improve *gut microbiome, intermittent fasting (IF), and time-restricted eating (TRE)* have been shown to improve insulin sensitivity by reducing fasting insulin levels and allowing cells to reset their metabolic processes.

As we discussed, you might consider several products that form the key to improved mitochondrial function and insulin sensitization, including *magnesium, berberine, chromium, Vitamin D_3, CoQ10, and PQQ.* Addressing *sarcopenia* is a vital part of an anti-aging strategy and I strongly recommend you incorporate it with the detailed treatments outlined in chapter 12. A few key things to remember here include *resistance training, creatine, proper protein intake, HMB, urolithin A, and ursolic acid supplements.*

For ALL my patients, regardless of age or health status, I target for a total cholesterol level less than 150 mg/dl and an LDL (bad cholesterol) level under 70 mg/dl. This can often be achieved without the use of drugs by adopting a whole-food, plant-based diet free of processed foods.

We explored how to take care of *systemic chronic inflammation (SCI) and gut health* in chapter 13. Chronic inflammation, low-grade yet impacting the entire body, is another primary driver of aging and age-related diseases. Therefore, I emphasize you should place a strong focus on reducing inflammation through nutrition, supplements, and regenerative therapies, all designed to protect your body at the cellular level. *Besides an anti-inflammatory diet, consider including metformin, low-dose naltrexone, colchicine, curcumin, boswellia, and tulsi tea.* I shared with you my simple personal recipe of *healthy herbal tea,* made by boiling water with some tulsi leaves, ginger, clove, and cinnamon sticks; and optionally topping the brew with honey and lemon.

As we discussed in that chapter, the *gut microbiome* plays a pivotal role in both metabolic insulin resistance and chronic inflammation. Imbalances in gut bacteria (dysbiosis) can be reversed with strategies like increasing dietary fiber to feed your healthy microbiome, taking triphala, consuming fermented foods (for example, yogurt, kefir, sauerkraut), and taking targeted probiotics to restore microbiome balance, improving insulin sensitivity.

5. Special Personalized Compounded Medicines

With guidance from an experienced physician, you can easily incorporate many of the compounded medicinal products, as they are readily available these days from compounding pharmacies. These compounded medicines can give you access to the latest in personalized, longevity-focused treatments. I strongly recommend ensuring that the pharmacy you or your physician use is *FDA-certified and based in the United States. You can verify this by checking with the pharmacy directly and checking with your state's pharmacy board.*

We talked about the research on the senolytic effects of rapamycin. Through careful compounding, we can create tailored formulations that allow for *intermittent, cyclical microdosing* (for example, 4–8 mg once a week, with a schedule of eight weeks on and eight weeks off.

Low-dose naltrexone (LDN) is an exciting, relatively unconventional therapy that's gaining a lot of attention in the world of autoimmune, anti-inflammation, and chronic illness treatment. The best way to use LDN is to start with a low dose (0.5 to 1.5 mg a day) and gradually increase it (up to 8 mg a day), allowing the body to adjust and maximize its immune-modulating benefits.

IV infusion therapies used as a once- or twice-monthly routine, or just intermittently with on and off schedules of few months each, are a great addition for many patients. I have found NAD+, as IV or subcutaneous route, to be a promising compounded product that has broad clinical application, and I incorporate this for many patients starting on VitalLife. You should consider IV glutathione as a compound that plays a critical role in detoxification, immune function, and cellular repair. Several medical spas now offer infusion therapies, such as longevity and immunity cocktails, glutathione, and NAD+ infusions. Make sure it is administered under the direct supervision of a physician.

6. Lifestyle Modifications

Lifestyle modifications are essential complements to the other modalities discussed above. As we explored in chapter 5, *studies on centenarians provide valuable insights about the role of lifestyle modifications for longevity*. These include nurturing meaningful social relationships, engaging in regular brain training, cultivating positive personality traits such as optimism and laughter, discovering your purpose, practicing gratitude, and embracing the act of giving.

The importance of lifestyle modifications cannot be overstated, which is why I have dedicated four entire chapters, 15 through 18, to exploring these in depth. Those chapters brought everything together, outlining the foundational daily habits necessary for lifelong health.

Chapter 15 emphasizes the cornerstone of any health journey: *incorporating a healthy nutritional plan*. I believe this is the most crucial factor in achieving long-term well-being. To begin, it's vital to eliminate key environmental toxins, that *unholy trinity* we talked about: smoking, excessive alcohol consumption, and poor dietary choices. Of particular importance is avoiding processed, ultra-processed, and deep-fried foods.

I strongly advocate for a *whole-food, plant-based diet*, a scientifically proven approach to optimizing health and longevity. For many, starting gradually may be more practical—perhaps trying one plant-based meal a day or adopting this diet for a couple of days each week. As a physician with decades of experience, I can confidently state that this dietary modification is nothing short of transformative. It stands as the most effective strategy to boost healthspan and not only prevent but also reverse diseases, including cardiovascular disease—the number one health-related killer worldwide. This dietary lifestyle is the cornerstone of achieving optimal health and longevity, holding the unparalleled potential to save countless lives and revolutionize global health. Its significance cannot be overstated.

Intermittent fasting and calorie restriction are also beneficial practices to incorporate. And don't forget to try the three simple recipes for healthy smoothies I included in that chapter, along with the tips I shared for naturally boosting your "inner Ozempic."

As we talked about in chapter 16, where we discussed *exercise*, I want you to focus on strength training to prevent and treat sarcopenia—loss of muscle mass and strength. Remember, it is important to have consistency, progressively increasing in resistance or weights, and allowing enough time for rest and recovery. In chapter 17 we talked about *herbs and supplements* for optimal cellular function. Some important ones to consider include fisetin, pentadecylic acid, rhodiola, NMN, and ashwagandha, among others.

Now, about the transformative power of *mindfulness and sound sleep*, as we discussed in chapter 18. Gratitude, service, charity, and calmer lifestyle go a long way to enhance both health and longevity. Establishing a good sleep hygiene routine is equally vital. Techniques such as meditation and yoga are powerful tools for fostering resilience, mental clarity, and emotional balance. Choose a simple mindfulness technique that resonates with you, such as *so hum* mantra mediation or body scan, and commit to it without any particular goal in mind. While the results may not be immediate, over time, those around you will notice a calmer, less stressed, more compassionate, emotionally balanced, productive, and level-headed version of yourself. And honestly, who wouldn't want that?

This detailed information about VitalLife guides you with a proactive, science-based, comprehensive approach to reach your goals of youthfulness, disease reversal, and longevity, empowering you to take charge of your health at every stage. Now, the journey continues with your own personalized 6-step program. I encourage you to take these insights and make them your own. Embrace this chance to invest in your future, and take the first step toward a vibrant, healthier life. Like a wise one said: *Life isn't about waiting for the storm to pass, life is about learning how to dance in the rain.* The transformation awaits, and it begins with your commitment today.

In the final chapter ahead, we'll explore the very essence of why you picked up this book—to fully embrace the journey of staying youthful for longer.

CHAPTER 20

Embracing a Brand-New You

> Man is so made that when anything fires his soul, impossibilities vanish.
> —Jean de La Fontaine, French poet (1621–1695)

> It isn't the mountains ahead to climb that wear you out; it's the pebble in your shoe.
> —Muhammad Ali, American professional boxer and social activist (1942–2016)

With everything you've learned in this book, you now have the knowledge to embark on your own journey of transformation. This program has already helped countless patients regain their youth, energy, and vitality—and it can do the same for you, only if you commit to it. This program isn't just about living longer; it's also about living better. Now *you have the tools to make that a reality.*

Your health is truly in your hands. As we've explored throughout this book, not only can symptoms or diseases be addressed, but even the aging process itself is not as inevitable as it may seem. The details of this program are here to help you unlock the vibrant, youthful energy that lies within you. This is your journey to a healthier, more fulfilling future.

Over the past many years, I've been privileged to guide patients from all walks of life who sought out to regain their health and reverse diseases. Across all of these experiences, one truth remains the same: *your body has an extraordinary ability to heal, rejuvenate, and thrive when given the right tools.* The principles you've learned in this book are the keys to unlocking that potential.

Finding a Reason Why

I'm reminded of a story a colleague, a family physician, shared with me some time ago. His patient, Martha, was a successful business owner in her mid-forties, managing four locations and living the demanding, stressful life so common among entrepreneurs. Like many, she was battling "diseases of abundance": obesity, diabetes, high blood pressure, and high cholesterol. Despite seeing multiple specialists and taking numerous medications, she struggled to make lasting progress, especially with her weight. For years, she would lose a few pounds only to gain them back, always explaining that she had "no time to exercise." Every three to six months, her doctors would counsel her, urging her to lose forty to fifty pounds to better manage her health.

As with many patients, Martha found it nearly impossible to achieve significant weight loss. Then, one day, my colleague was amazed to see her walk in forty-six pounds lighter. When he asked how she did it, she explained that she'd become disciplined, exercising an hour each morning before work, overhauling her diet completely, and consistently taking supplements. When he pressed her on what had finally motivated such a transformation after years of advice, she said, "Doc, about four months ago, my only son, who's just nineteen, was diagnosed with kidney failure. His doctors told him he needed a transplant to survive. As it turned out, I was the only match available for him, but the surgeon refused to proceed until I lose fifty pounds. He is my only son, so I had no choice, I had to do it. Now, we are scheduled for his transplant surgery in two weeks."

In my years of practice, I've seen this kind of transformation time and time again. Patients may be told to quit smoking for years without success, but a single ER visit with chest pain can be the spark that changes everything. *I truly believe that once pas-*

sion ignites our soul, we're capable of extraordinary deeds. Finding your "WHY" is the essential first step in any journey of transformation, especially one as impactful as the VitalLife program. *Your why is that inner motivation*—the reason that drives you past short-term fixes and sparks a true, lasting commitment to your health, especially when you feel you cannot carry on. In my experience, when patients *uncover a true, heartfelt purpose that resonates deeply*—whether it's to be more energized for their family or to reclaim a sense of strength and vitality—they are far more likely to stay the course.

With your purpose firmly in place, the knowledge you gained from this book will help bring your vision to life—empowering you not only to improve your health but to feel fully alive every day.

Knowledge Without Action Is Futile

All our dreams can come true, if we have the courage to pursue them.

—Walt Disney

We all dream about things that we would like to have or achieve, but for various reasons, we don't or are not able to take the required action to achieve what we dream. As we reach the conclusion of this book, I want to offer you more than just information—I want to inspire and empower you to act, *to act*. As a wise man once said, *"It's not what you know but what you do that truly matters."* Knowledge alone is powerless without action. It's not enough to understand what's possible—you must take that first step, make that commitment, and turn information into transformation. Real change happens when you channel what you know into deliberate, consistent action. *The key to progress lies not just in learning but in doing.*

> I truly believe that life is meant to be lived and not to be wasted on an endless—and ultimately futile—struggle to become the "master of the universe."

I know personally how working to make a living so often gets in the way of truly living life. I urge you to break free from this trap and begin your real journey today. The path to a younger, disease-free, more energetic you starts here, and it demands *consistency and discipline*. Because I've seen incredible transformations in my patients who committed to this journey, I'm confident that you can experience the same. The human body is capable of remarkable regeneration. By following the steps in this program as outlined, you are giving your body the very best chance to thrive, to live healthier longer. The journey toward health and longevity is one that requires commitment, but the rewards are immeasurable.

One thing I want you to take away is this: *you are in control.* The knowledge you've gained from this book has equipped you to make the choices that will dramatically impact the quality of your life. Whether you're in your thirties, fifties, or seventies, your body is ready to respond to the changes you make today. *It's never too late to start*, and the results are within your reach. I've seen patients who once thought they were too old or too far gone completely turn their lives around. With a few targeted, consistent efforts, they not only regained their health but found a new sense of purpose and vitality. *And while the journey isn't always easy, I can promise you it's worth it. Remember, you're not just investing in a longer life; you're investing in a life filled with energy, strength, and joy.*

Seeking *professional guidance* is crucial to making sure you stay on the right path. In my years of experience, the patients who succeeded most in their transformation were those who didn't do it alone. Having a team of experts who can help tailor this program to your unique needs—whether it's a nutritionist to adjust your nutrition plan, personal trainer to refine your exercise regimen, or an experienced physician introducing advanced regenerative therapies—makes all the difference. This is your journey, and you don't have to navigate it alone.

As you close this book, remember *this is not an ending, but the start of a new journey.* Picture yourself with the energy and focus you had ten, twenty, or even thirty years ago, waking up strong, engaged, and ready to embrace the day. What lies ahead is more than just extended time; it's a life filled with quality, connection, and fulfillment. Let the insights from this program guide you as you take charge of your health, your aging process, and your future.

This is your moment. The path to rejuvenation is in front of you, and the possibilities are endless. Your journey awaits—embrace it with open arms, and step into the vibrant life you deserve. I am sure by now you know I like great quotations that inspire and motivate. So, my dear friends, here is one more till we meet next, from Eleanor Roosevelt: *"The purpose of life is to live it, to taste experience to the utmost, to reach out eagerly and without fear for newer and richer experience."* I firmly believe that life is meant to be lived, not wasted on an endless—and ultimately futile—pursuit of becoming the "master of the universe".

I applaud you for embracing this journey and can't wait to see the transformation unfold, bringing you closer to the vibrant life you deserve.

Acknowledgments

I cannot imagine forging an unbeaten path, designing this unconventional VitalLife program, or writing this manuscript based on this program, without the steadfast encouragement and inspiration of so many remarkable people throughout my entire life. For this reason, I want to acknowledge not only those directly involved in this project but also the many others who have served as my North Star throughout my life.

First of all, I want to thank my patients and their families who entrusted me with their most precious asset—their health—I owe you my deepest gratitude. You have inspired me to pour my heart and soul into this work.

I borrow the timeless words from a beloved song: "You are my sunshine, my only sunshine; You make me happy when skies are gray." These words perfectly describe my beloved wife, Bina. She has stood by me through the highs and lows of my life, offering unwavering love, support, and belief in me—even when others would have walked away. Despite being long inflicted with this cruel illness called schizophrenia, Bina remains the most loving, gentle, kind, and compassionate soul I have ever known. More than that, she has been instrumental in the creation of this book. From reading those early, clunky drafts to preventing me from losing any more of what little hair I have left, she has been as vital to this project as I have. I truly couldn't have done it without you. To my wife of thirty-six years, Bina, I am endlessly grateful for your love and strength, which continue to illuminate my path.

To my parents, who are now with me in spirit, thank you for your unwavering love and guidance, for instilling in me the values of kindness and compassion that have shaped me as a healer. With deepest gratitude to my beloved sons, Kush and Neil, whose boundless curiosity, honest opinion, and love of life inspired every page of this book. Thank you both for always believing in me and encouraging my writing journey. You guys taught me the true meaning of wonder and unconditional love. You two are the heroes of my life.

Sir Isaac Newton once said, "If I have seen further, it is by standing on the shoulders of giants." I am profoundly grateful to the brilliant scientists, physicians, scholars, healers, and truth seekers who have shaped my thinking, inspired my work, and provided creative spark. These are my role models for excellence and serving humanity. Many are alive today, while others have moved on to their next adventure. Among them, I wish to thank and honor Socrates, Ralph Waldo Emerson, Rumi, Seneca, Nathan Pritikin, Tony Robbins, Dean Ornish, Jennifer Doudna, Napoleon Hill, Jane Goodall, Malcolm Gladwell, Bob Dylan, Shinya Yamanaka, Sir John Gurdon, Robert Lanza, Deepak Chopra, Elizabeth H. Blackburn, Yuval Noah Harari, David Brooks, Epictetus, Joseph Campbell, Oliver Sacks, Walter Gilbert, Will Durant, Thomas Friedman, and Siddhartha Mukherjee. Your insights have enriched my life and the lives of countless others.

Nothing great in life is ever done alone. This book has been a dream of mine for years, and now it is in your hands thanks to the extraordinary efforts of many. To my book editors, proofreader, designer, and publisher, I am deeply grateful for the guidance, expertise, and dedication, which made this book a reality against all odds. As famed NFL football coach Vince Lombardi once said, "Perfection is not attainable, but if we chase perfection, we can catch excellence." Together we tried to follow just that in this endeavor.

My sincere goal in writing this book has been to empower you with the knowledge and insights needed to transform your life. So, to you, the reader: thank you for joining me on this journey of discovery and empowerment with these transformative, nontraditional approaches to wellness and longevity. I offer you my best wishes as you get ready to embark on your journey for a new and younger you.

APPENDIX

Practical Resources for Improved Healthspan and Longevity

Dr. Hardesh Garg's Websites

VitalLifeProgram.com: To schedule an appointment with our clinic, explore blogs on the latest advancements in healthspan optimization, longevity, and regenerative medicine, and discover more about our current drug development programs.

Binacares.org: Non-profit to help patients suffering from neuropsychiatric illnesses.

The following list includes a wide variety of books, websites, videos, courses, research databases, and practical tools regarding regenerative and anti-aging health. Each resource is explained with its unique value and how to best use it for your optimal health journey.

—

NOTE: *This information is only provided to help readers. The author does not receive any financial incentives from any of the resources listed below.*

BOOKS

Lifespan: Why We Age and Why We Don't Have To, by David Sinclair, PhD: A groundbreaking book that explores genetic and biological mechanisms of aging and offers practical lifestyle interventions, including dietary changes and supplement use.

The Telomere Effect, by Dr. Elizabeth Blackburn and Dr. Elissa Epel: Discusses how lifestyle choices influence telomeres and biological aging.

The Longevity Diet, by Dr. Valter Longo: Outlines fasting and fasting-mimicking diet interventions for healthy aging. It provides practical dietary protocols for longevity.

Outlive: The Science & Art of Longevity, by Dr. Peter Attia: Comprehensive insights on metabolic health, nutrition, and exercise for longevity.

Healthy Aging, by Andrew Weil, MD: A holistic approach to longevity, covering mind-body balance. The book includes tips on diet, exercise, and mindfulness.

The Science and Technology of Growing Young, by Sergey Young: An overview of technological advancements in anti-aging.

The Circadian Code, by Dr. Satchin Panda: Explores how aligning lifestyle with circadian rhythms enhances health. Advises you to adjust your eating patterns for better health.

Super Human, by Dave Asprey: A guide to biohacking and advanced anti-aging techniques.

The Immunity Code, by Joel Greene: Focuses on optimizing immunity to promote longevity. Provides detailed protocols for gut health and immunity.

The Blue Zones Secrets for Living Longer, by Dan Buettner: Explores lifestyle habits from the world's longest-living populations. You can apply lessons from Blue Zones to improve longevity.

The End of Alzheimer's, by Dr. Dale Bredesen: Offers practical strategies for preventing cognitive decline. You can integrate brain-healthy habits into your daily routine.

Dr. Dean Ornish's Program for Reversing Heart Disease, by Dr. Dean Ornish: He is the first clinician to offer documented proof that heart disease can be halted, or even reversed, simply by changing your lifestyle.

Radical Longevity, by Ann Louise Gittleman: Explores anti-aging strategies, including detoxification and nutrition to improve healthspan.

Boundless, by Ben Greenfield: Covers biohacking techniques for optimizing health and longevity. Provides practical tips on sleep, exercise, and nutrition.

The Longevity Solution, by Dr. Jason Fun: Focuses on fasting and nutritional strategies for extending lifespan. Helps you to implement intermittent fasting protocols.

Ageless, by Andrew Steele: Explores scientific breakthroughs in longevity research.

Younger Next Year, by Chris Crowley and Dr. Henry Lodge: Provides actionable tips on exercise and lifestyle for longevity.

The Metabolic Approach to Cancer, by Dr. Nasha Winters: Focuses on metabolic health to prevent age-related diseases. You can optimize your diet and lifestyle to reduce disease risk.

WEBSITES

American Academy of Anti-Aging Medicine (www.a4m.com): Provides certifications, webinars, and research updates.

National Institute on Aging (https://www.nia.nih.gov): Offers research-backed articles on aging and longevity.

FoundMyFitness (https://www.foundmyfitness.com): Dr. Rhonda Patrick's platform for longevity science. Provides videos and podcasts.

Lifespan.io (www.lifespan.io): Funds longevity research and provides news updates. You can follow emerging therapies and clinical trials.

Mayo Clinic Center for Regenerative Medicine (https://www.mayo.edu): Shares updates on regenerative treatments. Great for the latest information to track clinical trials and new therapies.

Buck Institute for Research on Aging (https://www.buckinstitute.org): The first independent institute focused solely on aging. Provides its latest research papers.

Forks over Knives (https://www.forksoverknives.com): It empowers people to live healthier lives by changing the way the world understands nutrition. The title serves as a call to action: fight disease by changing what you eat, and you can avoid going under a surgeon's knife.

Longevity.Technology (https://www.longevity.technology): Covers news and innovations in longevity science. Keeps you updated on the latest trends.

One Meal a Day (OMD) (https://omdfortheplanet.com): Founded by Suzy Amis Cameron, this site supports and encourages eating at least one plant-based meal a day for your health and the planet's.

Healthline Anti-aging Hub (https://www.healthline.com): Provides practical tips and research-backed articles. Use it to implement daily habits for better health.

Healthline—Supplements Hub (https://www.healthline.com/nutrition): Healthline is one of the most popular health websites in the world. Their Supplements Hub offers evidence-based articles on a wide variety of supplements, including dosage guidelines, health benefits, and potential side effects.

Singularity Hub (https://www.singularityhub.com): Explores the future of technology and longevity. Good to follow updates on longevity tech.

Science Daily: Anti-aging News (https://www.sciencedaily.com): For breaking news about the latest discoveries in science and health from leading universities, scientific journals, and research organizations.

International Society for Stem Cell Research (ISSCR) (https://www.isscr.org): The ISSCR is the world's leading organization in stem cell science and regenerative medicine. Their website provides educational content for patients and researchers, along with ethical guidelines and updates on clinical trials.

Wake Forest Institute for Regenerative Medicine (WFIRM): WFIRM is a pioneer in regenerative medicine, particularly in 3D bioprinting, tissue engineering, and organ regeneration. The institute focuses on developing replacement tissues and organs to address medical needs.

National Institute of Health (NIH)—Regenerative Medicine (https://stemcells.nih.gov): This website offers comprehensive, research-backed information on stem cells, gene therapy, and tissue regeneration. It also provides updates on clinical trials and federal research initiatives.

InsideTracker Blog (https://www.insidetracker.com): Covers personalized health and biomarker tracking. Created by experts in aging and genetics from Tufts University and the Massachusetts Institute of Technology (MIT).

TruAge Test (TruDiagnostic.com): Biological test and DNA based insights for aging, nutrition, and more.

Galleri Test (https://www.galleri.com): This early-detection test can detect more than fifty kinds of cancer and determine the organ or tissue it originated in.

The Sleep Foundation (https://www.sleepfoundation.org): It is one of the most trusted online resources for sleep science, featuring evidence-based articles on topics like insomnia, sleep hygiene, and circadian rhythms.

Harvard University—Sleep and Health Education Gateway (UnderstandingSleep.org): It provides credible content about sleep disorders and disease management with reference material about sleep health that matters to you.

Examine.com (https://examine.com): It is one of the most trusted and comprehensive resources for science-backed information on supplements and nutrition.

NIH Office of Dietary Supplements (ODS) (https://ods.od.nih.gov): The National Institutes of Health (NIH) provides official, evidence-based information on dietary supplements. This website includes fact sheets, reports, and research on the safety and efficacy of various supplements.

VIDEOS

NOTE: *Most of these can be accessed on YouTube and by searching on Google.*

TED Talk: Dr. David Sinclair—Can We Reverse Aging: A concise overview of longevity science by a leading researcher in the field of aging.

Dr. Valter Longo on Fasting and Longevity: Advancing Healthspan and Longevity Innovation in Fasting-Mimicking Diet Research with Dr. Valter Longo. Many detailed interviews and webinars covering fasting protocols and their impact on extending lifespan. Can be found on YouTube and at https://createcures.org.

The Game Changers: A Netflix documentary about a plant-based diet for athletes. Documentary shows how elite athletes can achieve peak performance while following a vegan lifestyle. Showcases Novak Djokovic, Lewis Hamilton, Venus Williams, Jackie Chan, several Olympians, and others.

The Science of Longevity, by Dr. Peter Attia (TED Talk): Dr. Attia explains the difference between lifespan and healthspan. He highlights biomarkers and interventions that promote longevity and prevent chronic diseases.

The End of Alzheimer's, by Dr. Dale Bredesen (TEDx): Dr. Bredesen presents how to prevent and reverse cognitive decline through lifestyle changes, personalized nutrition, and hormone balance.

Rewire Your Brain for Longevity, by Dr. Joe Dispenza: This explores how thoughts, emotions, and meditation can influence genetic expression and longevity.

Huberman Lab Podcast: Dr. Andrew Huberman on Longevity: Covers cutting-edge insights on aging, brain health, and performance.

The Root Cause of Aging: by Dr. Aubrey de Grey (YouTube): A renowned gerontologist discusses the root causes of aging and potential solutions to reverse it.

The Longevity Film (documentary): Explores different cultures and their longevity secrets, highlighting lifestyle habits.

How Not to Die, by Dr. Michael Greger: Dr. Greger provides evidence-based advice on how a whole-food, plant-based diet can prevent chronic diseases and promote longevity.

How Diet and Lifestyle Affect Aging and Brain Function, by Dr. Rhonda Patrick: Rhonda Patrick, PhD, discusses how diet can affect DNA damage and initiates cancer.

Why Enhancing Metabolic Health Could Be the Key to Preventing Alzheimer's Disease, by Dr. David Perlmutter: Explores the relationship between diet, inflammation, and cognitive longevity.

Imagining the Future: The Transformation of Humanity, by Peter Diamandis (TEDx LA): Explores innovations in biotechnology and anti-aging therapies that may redefine aging.

Longevity & Biohacking, by Ben Greenfield: A comprehensive video series on biohacking techniques to improve longevity and vitality.

Unlocking the Secrets of Longevity with Dr. David Sinclair (YouTube): *Longevity by Design* host Dr. Gil Blander speaks with Dr. David Sinclair, a professor of genetics at Harvard Medical School, about the science behind aging and how we can extend both lifespan and healthspan.

Hormone Health and Longevity, by Dr. Sara Gottfried: A video interview focusing on how hormones play a role in slowing the aging process.

The Biology of Aging, by Khan Academy: A free video series diving deep into the biological processes of aging.

Reversing Aging by Big Think: A compilation of interviews with experts discussing cutting-edge anti-aging science.

Hyperbaric Oxygen Therapy for Longevity, by Dr. Shai Efrati: Dr. Efrati shares research on hyperbaric oxygen therapy (HBOT) and its impact on telomere length and cognitive function.

Biomarkers for Longevity, by Dr. Gil Blander: Dr. Blander emphasizes the importance of personalized biomarker testing for longevity.

WEBSITES FOR RESEARCH FOR ADVANCED LEARNING

PubMed (https://pubmed.ncbi.nlm.nih.gov/): A comprehensive database from the National Library of Medicine of peer-reviewed research articles on aging and regenerative medicine. You can search for studies on specific topics like cellular senescence, telomeres, and stem cells.

ClinicalTrials.gov: A database of past and ongoing clinical trials, including those focused on regenerative therapies and anti-aging interventions. Track ongoing trials and consider participating in relevant studies.

ResearchGate: A platform connecting researchers with access to papers and collaborations across various fields. Follow top researchers in longevity science and stay updated on their work.

Google Scholar: A powerful tool to find academic papers and research studies on anti-aging and regenerative medicine. Use advanced search filters to find specific studies relevant to your interests.

Longevity Database by Lifespan.io: A curated collection of longevity-related research papers, news, and updates. Explore emerging therapies and their clinical evidence to stay informed.

Aging Cell Online: One of the leading journals covering the biology of aging and longevity research. Stay updated on groundbreaking studies and their practical applications.

Nature Aging Online: A scientific journal that covers advancements in longevity and aging-related research. Read reviews and papers to stay informed about the latest findings.

ScienceDirect: A database of peer-reviewed journals, including articles on regenerative medicine and aging. Access full-text research papers to deepen your understanding of longevity science.

BioRxiv: A preprint server for biology research, including cutting-edge studies on aging, before formal publication. It is operated by the renowned Cold Spring Harbor Laboratory in Laurel Hollow, New York.

SpringerLink: Provides access to journals and books on health sciences and aging research. You can search for longevity and anti-aging research papers for detailed insights.

PLOS Biology Online: An open-access journal covering topics like genetics, aging, and regenerative medicine. Access cutting-edge research articles for free.

JAMA Network Online: The *Journal of the American Medical Association*, a collection of peer-reviewed medical journals covering various health topics, including aging. Stay current with clinical research on aging and longevity.

The Lancet Healthy Longevity Online (https://www.thelancet.com/journals/lanhl/home): A British medical journal focused on aging-related health issues and interventions. Read the latest research on population health and longevity.

Cell Metabolism Online: A journal that explores the connection between metabolism and aging.

Trends in Molecular Medicine Online: A journal covering breakthroughs in molecular research related to aging. Read detailed reviews and original research articles.

Frontiers in Aging Neuroscience Online: Covers research on aging and its impact on the brain. Explore topics on neuroplasticity and cognitive decline prevention.

Nature Reviews Molecular Cell Biology Online: Focuses on cellular and molecular mechanisms of aging. Keep up with the latest scientific findings.

eLife Online: An open-access journal that covers life sciences research, including aging and longevity.

The Journals of Gerontology Online: A series of journals focusing on the biology, psychology, and social aspects of aging. It dives into research that explores the multifactorial nature of aging.

PRACTICAL TOOLS AND APPS

Smartwatches for health data: Good for measuring health metrics and performance data. Most common are Apple Watch, Fitbit, Garmin, Spade & Co., Google Pixel watch, Garmin Forerunner.

InsideTracker: A company founded with a team of experts from MIT and Harvard and Tufts Universities. Provides personalized biomarker tracking and longevity recommendations.

FreeStyle Libre3 by Abbott: A continuous glucose monitoring (CGM) system that allows people to track their blood sugar levels in real time.

WHOOP: Wearable technology for tracking recovery, sleep, and strain. Utilize data to optimize your training and recovery routines.

Headspace: A mindfulness app to reduce stress and promote longevity through meditation. Practice daily meditation to improve your mental and emotional health.

MyFitnessPal: A comprehensive food tracking app to monitor your dietary intake. Track your diet and adjust your eating habits for longevity-focused nutrition.

Calm: A mindfulness and sleep app to improve recovery and reduce stress levels. Use meditation sessions and sleep stories to enhance your rest and recovery.

AmritYoga.com: An authentic yoga center and nonprofit ashram It offers online courses and certifications in yoga, yoga nidra, and yoga therapy, as well as health retreats.

Oura Ring: A smart wearable that tracks sleep, activity, and readiness. Adjust your routines based on data insights to optimize your recovery.

KardiaMobile EKG Monitors: FDA-cleared to detect AFib and allows detailed reporting on your heart data.

Zero Fasting App: Tracks fasting routines and provides insights on metabolic health. Use it to implement various fasting protocols for health and longevity.

Cronometer: An advanced nutrition tracking tool that tracks micronutrients. Helps you ensure you're getting essential vitamins and minerals to optimize your diet.

Pillow App: A sleep-tracking app that provides insights on your sleep patterns. You can use the insights from your data to optimize your sleep hygiene.

HRV4Training: Tracks heart rate variability to assess recovery and readiness for physical activity. Good to use your HRV data to fine-tune your exercise and recovery plans.

NutraCheck: A comprehensive food diary and calorie counter app to make sure you're meeting your nutritional goals.

Muse Headband: A wearable device that provides real-time feedback on brain activity during meditation. Use the feedback to improve your meditation practice and reduce stress.

Strava: A fitness tracking app for running, cycling, and other physical activities. Track your workouts and monitor your progress over time to optimize physical fitness for longevity.

Wellue O2Ring: A wearable device that tracks blood oxygen levels, heart rate, and body movements while you sleep.

The EMAY SleepO2 Pro Sleep Apnea Monitor: A personal sleep apnea monitor for home use. The wrist-worn device monitors blood oxygen saturation and heart rate while you sleep.

INDEX

4-hydroxy-trans-2-nonenal (HNE), 253
5-Methoxy-N,N-Dimethyltryptamine (5-MeO-DM), 152

A

AA/EPA Ratio, 94
abdominal fat, 59, 90, 195, 198, 207
adaptive immunity, 56–57
addiction, 144, 151, 160, 162–163, 165–166
addiction recovery, 165
adenosine triphosphate (ATP), 60
adult stem cells (ASCs), 118
advanced anti-inflammatory protocol, 244
advanced glycation end products (AGEs), 255
advanced peptides, 198–199
aerobic exercise, 285, 287
afternoon green detox smoothie, 274
aging
  biological, 52–54, 73
  disease, 65–83
  hallmarks of, 52–54
  immune cell theory of, 56–57
  mechanisms, 20, 55, 62, 68
  metabolic insulin resistance theory of, 59–60
  mitochondrial energy theory of, 60–63
  senescent cells in, 55–56
  Systemic Chronic Inflammation (SCI), 57–59
  theories of, 54–64
  vascular, 74
  VitalLife model of, 70–72
  zombie cells, 55
aging skin, 217
Aging Triad, 39–40, 67–71, 40, 189–190, 319, 326–327
alcohol abuse, 251
allergy testing, 95
allogeneic stem cells, 117
Alpert, Richard, 145
alpha-lipoic acid (ALA), 194
Altman, Sam, 27
Altos Labs, 26
Alzheimer's disease, 14, 159–160, 253
Amazon, 26
Amazonian indigenous medicine, 292
American and Canadian Diabetes Associations, 266
American Botanical Council, 297
American ginseng, 197
American Heart Association, 91
amyloid protein, 14
amylopectin, 202
anabolic resistance, 81
Ancient CHamoru (or Chamorro) medicine, 292
angiogenesis, 123
angioplasty, 17, 80, 243
anti-aging hormone, 184. *see also* DHEA (dehydroepiandrosterone)
anti-aging/youthfulness, 155, 166
  hyperbaric oxygen therapy (HBOT), 108–110
  medical technologies for, 110
  ozone therapy for, 107–108
  parabiosis for, 105–107
  protocols, 4, 24, 30, 184
antibiotics, 254
anti-inflammatory
  diet, 209–210

protocol, 116, 244, 322
anxiety, 159, 216, 226–227, 237–238, 244, 253, 267–268, 284, 300, 303
apoptosis, 62, 224–225
Archives of Internal Medicine, 190
aromatase inhibitors (AIs), 177
aromatization, 177
arthritis, 127
artificial intelligence, 26, 28, 31
artificial sweeteners, 256
ashwagandha, 213, 220, 292, 295
Association of Tennis Professionals (ATP), 8
atherosclerosis, 14, 17, 66, 68–70, 74–80, 211–212, 253
athletic performance, 43
attention deficit hyperactivity disorder (ADHD), 268
autologous stem cells, 117
autophagy, 53, 224
awareness and intentionality, 270
Ayurveda, 7, 207, 214, 291–292

B

bacopa, 294
bacterial endotoxins, 58
balance and flexibility exercises, 287–288
balance drills, 288
Bell, Kristen, 150
Berberine, 194, 279, 326
beta-hydroxy-beta-methyl butyrate (HMB), 200, 202
Bezos, Jeff, 26–27
Binacares.org, 341
biohacking, 9
bioidentical hormones, 237
biological age/aging, 13, 73, 89
   vs. chronological age, 18–20
biomarker assessment/tests, 87–96, 188, 205
   for personalized plan, 322–323
bitter melon, 197
blood
   tests, 95
   transfusions, 105–107
Blue Zone diet, 264
Blue Zones Project, 50
body-mass index (BMI), 90, 267
body scan, 307–308
bodyweight exercises, 286
bonding hormone, 183. see also love hormone
"bone-on-bone" disease, 129
boost energy levels, 123
boost immune health, 122
BPC-157 (Wolverine peptide), 186–187
brain
   active, 51
   health, 42
brain-derived neurotrophic factor (BDNF), 158, 160, 284
brain health and cognitive function, 284
brain health and mental well-being, 216
branched-chain amino acid (BCAA), 200
Bremelanotide. see PT-141
Brin, Sergey, 28
British Medical Journal, 267
brown adipose tissue (BAT), 197
Bryant, Kobe, 115

C

C3 and C4 complements, 93
calorie-dense diet, 245
calorie-dense food, 246
Campbell, T. Colin, 79
cardiologists as proxies, 17
cardiovascular disease, 14
cardiovascular health, 123, 283

carrageenan, 280
cellular feedback loop, 67–69
cellular health, 103
cellular health and mitochondria, 283
cellular rejuvenation, 38–39
cellular senescence, 53, 99
Celsus, Aulus Cornelius, 76
centenarians
  defined, 40
  lessons from, 41, 49–52
  studies of, 282
Chan, Priscilla, 28
charity, 51–52
chemical additives, 254–255
chestnut rose, 105
China Study, 78
chromium, 194, 201, 279, 326
chronic diseases, 42
  and cancers, 266–267
  silent progression of, 14–15
chronic inflammation, 39–40, 53, 68, 99, 265
  diagnostic testing, 92–94
chronic inflammation markers, 323
chronic joint/neck/low back pain, 131
chronic pain, 4, 7, 99, 111, 125, 129–131, 134, 164–166, 212, 226, 229, 308, 324
chronological age, 13, 18–20
  vs. biological age, 18–20
cinnamon, 197
Cleveland Clinic, 76–77, 248
clogged arteries, 77
cloves, 214
coenzyme Q10 (CoQ10), 194, 295
cognition, 37
cognitive decline, 159–160
cognitive function assessments, 91
colchicine, 40, 68, 212, 228, 326,
Colchicum autumnale plant, 212

cold exposure and thermogenesis, 197
complete blood count (CBC), 95
complex regional pain syndrome (CRPS), 164
compounded hormones and peptides, 235–240
  hormones and peptides for men, 236–237
  hormones and peptides for women, 237–239
compounded oral ketamine for microdosing protocol, 226–228
Confucius, 1
consciousness, 145–148
consistency, 289
continuous glucose monitors (CGMs), 90
Controlled Substances Act, 154
cookie-cutter approach, 171–172, 175
cornerstone of metabolic health, 195
cornerstone of muscle health, 200
Coronary heart disease (CHD), 78
cosmetic medicine, 128
COVID, 9, 42, 109
C-reactive protein (CRP), 211, 213
creatine, 202
CRISPR gene-editing, 31
cryotherapy, 112
curcumin, 197, 213, 279, 292, 294, 327
Curry, Steph, 115
cyclical regimen, 225
cycling, 287

D

dancing/low-impact aerobics classes, 287
dasatinib, 104
da Vinci, Leonardo, 24–25, 47
deep breathing exercises, 307
de Jiménez, Huautla, 145

de León, Juan Ponce, 22–23, 25
Deming, W. Edwards, 87
deoxyribonucleic acid (DNA), 31
depression, 159
DHEA (dehydroepiandrosterone), 184
Diabetes Care, 266
diet, 314
differentiation, 116
Dimethyltryptamine (DMT), 152
disease progression, 11, 15, 17, 58, 62, 94, 99, 122
diseases of abundance, 258–261, 332
DNA, 61
   methylation, 38, 53, 89, 323
   tests, 87–96
DNA methylation biological age tests, 323
Drucker, Peter, 87
drug-for-symptom approach, 16, 18
Dysbiosis, 53, 214–217

E

Ebstein, Wilhelm, 68
Einstein, Albert, 301
Electrical Muscle Stimulation (EMS), 112–113
Ellison, Larry, 27
embracing gratitude, 303
embryonic stem cells (ESCs), 117, 118
Emerson, Ralph Waldo, 65
emotional disorders, 162, 165
emotional well-being, 41, 51, 132, 141, 144, 153, 167, 183–184, 240, 252, 281–285, 289, 302, 308. *see also* well-being
environmental and ethical benefits, 268
environmental pollutants, 255
environmental toxins tests, 94–95
environment shape aging, 63–64

EPIC-Oxford study, 249
epidemic of loneliness in America, 310–311
epigenetics, 63–64
   alteration, 53
   modification, 63
erectile dysfunction (ED), 37, 128, 130–132
   treatments for, 132, 134–135
Erythrocyte Sedimentation Rate (ESR), 93
Esselstyn, Caldwell Jr., 191
estrogen, 238
estrogen blockers, 177–178, 236
evidence-based support, 196
exercise for strength and vitality, 281–290
   multifactorial challenge, 285–290
   for optimal aging, 285
   promotes both longevity and healthspan, 283–285
   for sarcopenia and aging, 285–290
exosome infusions, 120–121
exosomes, 19
exosomes and extracellular vesicles (EVs), 119

F

favor consistency over perfection, 270
fenugreek, 196–197
fermented foods, 279
Ferriss, Tim, 150
ferritin, 93
fiber-rich nutrition, 201
fibrinogen, 93
fisetin, 104, 293
flexibility and balance, 285
focused attention meditation, 306
follicle-stimulating hormone (FSH), 89, 178
Food and Drug Administration (FDA), 101, 154

food as medicine, 5
foods to avoid, 272
Fountain of Youth Archaeological Park, 23
Freeman, Morgan, 150
Frost, Robert, 12
fruits and vegetables, 279
functional medicine, 9

G
Galen, 24
Galleri, 91
Galleri cancer detection, 38
genetic cancer screening, 91
genomic instability, 52
GLP-1 (glucagon-like peptide-1), 278–279
glutathione, 234–235, 293
Glycosylated Acute-Phase Proteins (GlycA), 93
gonadorelin, 178, 237
gonadotropin-releasing hormone (GnRH), 178
grip strength test, 92
growth hormone (GH), 82, 183, 186
growth hormone–releasing hormone (GHRH), 172
guduchi *(Tinospora cordifolia)*, 294
Gurdon, John, 106
gut-associated lymphoid tissue (GALT), 215
gut-brain axis, 216
gut dysbiosis, 59–60, 62, 75, 189, 205, 216
gut health, 214–217
gut microbiome, 193, 210
gut-muscle axis, 201

H

hair and facial cosmetic rejuvenation, 133–134
hair loss, 128
hair tests, 95, 96
Handler, Chelsea, 150
health
  holistic approach to, 5
  money and, 29–30
healthspan, 13
  defined, 20
  vs. lifespan, 20–21
  optimization, 20, 21
healthy aging, 37
healthy eating, tips to, 273–274
heart and cardiovascular health, 216
heart disease, 77–81
heart health, 266
heavy metals, 255
heavy metal testing, 94
hematological (blood) tests, 91
hematopoietic stem cells, 118
herbal medicine, 219
herbs, 279
herbs and supplements, 314
high-fiber content in plant-based diet, 262–264
high-fiber foods, 279
high-intensity interval training (HIIT), 195, 288–289
highly processed foods, 280
high-sensitivity C-reactive protein (hs-CRP), 90, 93
high-sugar and refined carbohydrate foods, 280
hippocampus, 107, 156, 158, 159
Hippocrates, 24, 204
Hofmann, Albert, 143
holistic medicine, 9
Holy basil, 197, 213, 220, 294
Homeostasis Model Assessment for Insulin Resistance (HOMA-IR), 90
Hopkins, Johns, 149, 150, 156

hormonal and metabolic
    assessment, 170
hormonal and peptide
    imbalance, 170
hormonal changes, 82
hormonal levels, 89
hormonal optimization, 19, 39
hormones
    defined, 171
    growth hormone (GH), 183
    love, 172, 183, 237, 311
    and peptide optimization,
        325–326
    thyroid, 184–185
hormone dehydroepiandrosterone
    (DHEA), 89
hormone optimization, 169–187, 201
    comprehensive, 171–173, 182–187
    testosterone optimization therapy
        (TOT), 173–178
Hormone Optimization Therapy
    (HOT), 179, 182
    side effects and precautions of,
        181–182
    in women, 179–182
hormone replacement therapy
    (HRT), 179, 182
human chorionic gonadotropin
    (HCG), 178, 236–237
human growth hormone
    (HGH), 183
Human Longevity, 27
hyperbaric oxygen therapy (HBOT),
    108–110
hyperpermeability, 58
hypoactive sexual desire disorder
    (HSDD), 239

I

Ikaria, Greece, 50
Ikigai, 50
immortality, 1

immune cell theory, 56–57
immune function testing, 95–96
immune health, 284
immune system, 27, 40, 48, 58, 202,
    207–208, 210, 213, 223, 228–229,
    252, 283, 310, 312
immunity, 36–37, 42
    adaptive, 56–57
    and disease prevention, 215–216
    innate, 56–57
immunoglobulin E (IgE), 95
immunosenescence, 56–57
improve cognitive function, 123
improved gut health, 267
improve metabolic function,
    121–122
induced pluripotent stem cells
    (iPSCs), 118
inflammaging, 55, 57–59, 211
inflammation, 36–37
    diseases, 42
    reduce, 103
inflammatory bowel disease
    (IBD), 213
infrared therapy, 110–111
innate immunity, 56–57
inner healing power, 8
insulin, 16
insulin-like growth factor-1 (IGF-1),
    82, 201
insulin resistance, 14, 57, 59–61,
    67–73, 90, 100
insulin sensitivity and metabolic
    health, 265–266
intercellular communication, 53
interleukin-6 (IL-6), 82, 93–94, 211
intermittent dosing protocols,
    166, 227
intermittent fasting, 260–261
intermittent fasting and time-
    restricted eating, 193
intermittent microdosing, 225

Index

intravenous exosome infusions, 122–124
intravenous (IV) infusions of stem cells, 120–125
intravenous (IV) infusion therapies, 230–232, 328
intravenous (IV) placental stem cell infusions, 121–122
ipamorelin, 198

J

Jobs, Steve, 149
Johns Hopkins Medicine, 297
Johnson, Bryan, 97–98
Journal of Clinical Nutrition, 191
Journal of the American Medical Association *(JAMA)*, 79

K

Kennedy International Airport, 34
ketamine, 152–153, 163–168, 325
kykeon, 143

L

leaky gut, 58, 214–217
Leary, Timothy, 145
LED light therapy, 111
Life, 145
Life Biosciences, 27
lifespan, 13
  defined, 20
  healthspan *vs.*, 20–21
lifestyle modifications, 328–330
light-emitting diodes (LED), 111
lipopolysaccharides (LPS), 58
Lipoprotein-Associated Phospholipase A2 (Lp-PLA2), 93
Little White House, 29
living in present moment, 308
L-leucine, 200
localized autologous
  bone marrow stem cell treatments, 129–130
  fat-derived stem cell treatments, 130–131
localized platelet-rich plasma (PRP) therapy, 127–128
localized/targeted exosome treatments, 132–136
Loma Linda, California, 50
longevity, 42
  and healthy aging, 216–217
  mysteries of, 54–64
  and youthful energy, 265
Loneliness, epidemic of, 310–311
love hormone, 172, 183, 237, 311
low-calorie diet, 259–260
low-dose naltrexone (LDN), 211–212, 228–229, 327
low testosterone *(Low-T)*, 173. *see also* testosterone deficiency
luteinizing hormone (LH), 89, 178, 237
lysergic acid diethylamide (LSD), 143, 152

M

machines, 287
macrophages, 75
magnesium, 194, 201, 233, 273, 279, 326
major depressive disorder (MDD), 159
Manning, Peyton, 115
mantra meditation, 306
Mayo Clinic, 297
medical conditions improvement, 41–43
medical technological devices/ MedTech, 92
medications, 210–212
medicine. *see also* regenerative medicine/therapies

Amazonian indigenous, 292
Ancient CHamoru (or Chamorro), 292
cosmetic, 128
food as, 5
functional, 9
herbal, 219
holistic, 9
modern, 5, 20, 143, 145, 150, 156, 213, 292
personalized, 40
sports, 128
traditional, 15–18
traditional herbal, 196–197
Medisolare, 7, 207, 214, 291, 292
meditation techniques, 306
Mediterranean cultures, 246
MedTech. *see* medical technological devices
melatonin, 185, 295
Memorial Sloan Kettering Cancer Center (MSKCC), 297
memory hormone, 185
mental health, 267–268
mental illnesses, 42–43
mesenchymal stem cells (MSCs), 118, 121, 129–130
metabolic dysfunction, 58–59
metabolic endotoxemia, 58
metabolic health, 123
metabolic health and weight regulation, 216
metabolic insulin resistance theory, 39–40, 59–60, 99
metabolic medications, 196
metabolic regulators, 184–185. *see also* thyroid hormones
metabolic syndrome, 56, 59, 192, 265
metabolism, 188–203
  advanced natural compounds, 194–195
  advanced peptides, 198–199
  cold exposure and thermogenesis, 197
  combat mitochondrial dysfunction, 191–199
  cornerstone of metabolic health, 195
  detoxification, 192
  gut microbiome, 193
  helpers, 194–195
  insulin resistance, 189–199
  nutrition as catalyst for change, 192–193
  overview, 188–189
  practical strategies, 191–199
  role of the mitochondria, 189–191
  sarcopenia, 199–203
  stress management and restful sleep, 195–196
  timeless remedies for, 196–197
  traditional herbal medicine, 196–197
metformin, 40, 194, 196, 211, 227–228, 327
methylenedioxymethamphetamine (MDMA), 152–154, 159
microbiome, 214–217
microdose lithium orotate, 293
microdosing, 166, 227
microneedling with exosomes, 133
micronized progesterone, 180
microplastics and nanoplastics, 256
mind-body exercises, 285
mindfulness, 270
mindfulness and restful sleep, 299–315
  epidemic of loneliness in America, 310–311
  fundamentals, 302–305
  sleep hygiene, 311–315
  techniques for, 305–308
  technological tools in, 308–309

mindfulness meditation, 306
mitochondria, 53
mitochondrial cells, 60
mitochondrial damage, 61–62, 198
mitochondrial dysfunction, 39–40, 53, 60, 61–62, 68, 82, 99
mitochondrial energy theory of, 60–63
mitochondrial function, 91
mitophagy, 194
Mitopure, 194
modern medicine, 5, 20, 143, 145, 150, 156, 213, 292
mood, 37
morning smoothie, 274
multipotent stem cells, 118. *see also* adult stem cells (ASCs)
muscle mass, 37
muscle mass and bone density, 283
muscle regeneration, 123
musculoskeletal health, 134
Musk, Elon, 150
mycotoxins, 255
mycotoxin testing, 95

N

NAD+, 201, 227, 231, 232–235, 324, 328
Nadal, Rafael, 115
Naltrexone, low-dose (LDN), 211–212, 228–229
National Center for Complementary and Integrative Health (NCCIH), 296
National Football League, 8
National Institute on Aging, 225
natural growth hormone, 186
near-infrared therapy, 110–111
neurogenesis, 156–160
    diseases impacted by, 158–160
    psychedelics role in, 158
neuroplasticity, 155, 156–160

diseases impacted by, 158–160
psychedelics role in, 158
New England Journal of Medicine, 76, 190
Nicklaus, Jack, 115
nicotinamide mononucleotide (NMN), 233, 293
Nicoya, Costa Rica, 50
Nietzsche, Friedrich, 47
NIH Office of Dietary Supplements, 296
Nixon, Richard, 154
N-methyl-D-aspartate (NMDA), 164
nonsteroidal anti-inflammatory drugs (NSAIDs), 211
nurture meaningful relationships, 50–51
nutrient-dense diet, 50, 245
nutrient-dense foods, 192
nutrient sensing, 53

O

Okinawa, Japan, 50
    Okinawa Centenarian Study, 50, 249, 282
    Okinawa Research Center for Longevity Science, 50
omega-3 fatty acids, 194, 201, 209, 279, 295
optimizing protein intake, 200
oral estrogen, 181
organ-specific tests, 91
Ornish, Dean, 191
Osler, William, 1
oxidative phosphorylation, 60
oxidative stress tests, 89
oxLDL, 75
oxytocin, 172, 177, 183–184, 237–239, 311, 325
oxytocin nasal spray, 237
Ozempic (semaglutide), 278
ozone therapy, 107–108

P

parabiosis, 105–107
patient-centered approaches, 9
peak performance tests, 91–92
pentadecylic acid, 293, 329
peptides, defined, 171
peptides optimization, 39, 186–187
perfluoroalkyl substances (PFAS), 255
perinatal stem cells, 118–119
personal invitation, 9–11
personalized assessment/testing, 38, 87–96
personalized medicines, 40
personalized protocols, 102, 113, 115–116, 357
pesticides, 254
pesticide testing, 94–95
PGA Tour, 8
pharmaceutical compounding, 222–223
philosopher's stone, 24
Phthalates and Bisphenol A (BPA) testing, 95
physical and emotional well-being, 132
pilates, 288
placental/umbilical stem cell infusions, 120
plant-based diet, 51, 243–280
   "all-you-can-eat" diet, 271–274
   diets, 246–250
   diseases of abundance, 258–261
   high-fiber content in, 262–264
   learned behavior, 268–271
   Ozempic (semaglutide), 278–280
   proven benefits of, 265
   proven health benefits, 261–268
plant-based lifestyle, 244, 270, 271–274
plant-based milk, 262
plasmapheresis, 102–104
plastics and packaging chemicals, 255
platelet-rich plasma (PRP), 116, 125, 127–128, 131–134
pluripotent stem cells, 117. *see also* embryonic stem cells (ESCs)
polycyclic aromatic hydrocarbons (PAHs), 253, 256
poor diet, 251
positive mindset, 51
post-traumatic stress disorder (PTSD), 43, 144, 151–155, 159, 163, 165, 226, 322, 324
prebiotic foods, 218
pregnenolone, 185. *see also* memory hormone
preservatives, 255
Prince Harry, 149
Pritikin, Nathan, 191
probiotic-rich foods, 218
processed and ultra-processed foods, 257–258
progesterone, 39–40, 170, 180–182, 185, 237, 238
progressive overload, 289
promote tissue repair, 121
protect against insulin resistance, 263
proteins, 279
proteostasis dysfunction, 53
P-shots, 128, 132
psilocybin, 138–140, 142–144, 149–156, 158–160, 162–163, 324
psilocybin (natural), 151–152
psychedelic-assisted therapies, 161
psychedelic renaissance, 150
psychedelics, 137–168, 324
   consciousness, 145–148
   convergence of three transcendental states, 145–148
   current research with, 151–153
   diseases impacted by, 155–156

journeys of rich and famous, 149–151
ketamine, 163–168
legal status and current state of approval of, 153–154
magic mushroom, 161–163
neuroplasticity and neurogenesis, 156–160
role in health and longevity, 163–168
role in neurogenesis, 158
role in neuroplasticity, 158
transcendent mind, 140–142
use since ancient times, 142–145
PT-141, 39, 172, 186, 237, 239
pterostilbene, 104, 296
pulsed electromagnetic field therapy (PEMF), 111
Pyrroloquinoline quinone (PQQ), 195, 293

Q

quercetin, 104, 194, 213, 296

R

Ram Dass, 145
rapamycin, 105, 224–226
reactive oxygen species (ROS), 61
real healthcare, 21
reduce systemic inflammation, 121
reframing mind, 271
regenerative medicine/therapies, 30, 38–39, 42–43, 54, 83, 99, 115–117, 126, 134–135, 189, 319, 324, 327, 334
   cellular inflammation, 99
   current, 101–113
   cutting-edge, 19
   impact on diseases, 100–101
   power of, 97–113
   principles, 99–100
   senolytics, 104–105
   stem cell infusions, 120
   therapeutic plasma exchange (TPE), 102–104
Renaissance period, 24
renewed energy/recovery, 36
research-backed compounds for muscle function, 201–203
resistance bands, 286
rest and recovery, 289
resveratrol, 104, 194, 213, 292, 294
Retro Biosciences, 27
rhodiola, 294
Robbins, Tony, 115
Rodgers, Aaron, 149
Rogan, Joe, 150
Ronaldo, Cristiano, 115
Roosevelt, Franklin D., 29
Ross, American Russell, 76

S

saliva tests, 95
Salk, Jonas, 97
sarcopenia, 37, 81–83, 199–203
   additional tips for preventing, 289
   prevent and alleviate, 286
Sardinia, Italy, 50
saturated and trans fats, 280
selective estrogen receptor modulators (SERMs), 177
selective serotonin reuptake inhibitors (SSRIs), 164
self-renewal, 116
Semax, 198
semi-fasting, 260–261
senescence, 42
senescence-associated secretory phenotype (SASP), 55
senescent cells, 27, 55–56
senolytic drugs, 56
senolytics, 19, 104–105

sermorelin, 186, 198, 229–230, 237, 239, 277
sexual health, 37, 134–136
Shaw, George Bernard, 22
short-chain fatty acids (SCFAs), 215–216, 218
silent progression, 14–15
Sinatra, Frank Albert, 12
sleep, 311
   environment, 313
   hygiene, 311–315
   routine, 313
   quality, 312–313
   -wake cycle, 185
   well, 51
smoking, 251
social connections, 284–285
soluble fibers, 263
Spare (Prince Harry), 149
spiritual awakening, 140, 144
sports medicine, 128
Stanford University School of Medicine, 297
statins, 17
stem cells
   adult stem cells (ASCs), 118
   allogeneic, 117
   autologous, 117
   chronic joint/neck/low back pain, 131
   described, 116–119
   embryonic stem cells (ESCs), 117, 118
   exhaustion, 53
   and exosomes, 114–136
   hair and facial cosmetic rejuvenation, 133–134
   hematopoietic, 118
   induced pluripotent stem cells (iPSCs), 118
   intravenous exosome infusions, 122–124
   intravenous (IV) infusions, 120–125
   intravenous (IV) placental stem cell infusions, 121–122
   localized autologous bone marrow stem cell treatments, 129–130
   localized autologous fat-derived stem cell treatments, 130–131
   localized platelet-rich plasma (PRP) therapy, 127–128
   localized/targeted exosome treatments, 132–136
   localized/targeted procedures, 125–126
   mesenchymal stem cells (MSCs), 118
   musculoskeletal health, 134
   overview, 114–116
   perinatal, 118–119
   safety and effectiveness of IV, 125
   sexual health, 134–136
   treatments for erectile dysfunction (ED), 132
stimulate skin rejuvenation, 123
strength, 37
   exercises, 210
   training, 285, 286
streptomyces hygroscopicus, 224
stress management, 210, 313–314
stress management and restful sleep, 195–196
supplements and herbs, 213–214, 279, 291–298
symphony of regeneration, 8
synthetic progestins, 180
systemic chronic inflammation (SCI), 204–221
   anti-inflammatory diet, 209–210
   dysbiosis, 214–217
   exercise and mindfulness, 210
   gut health, 214–217
   gut microbiome, 210

Index

interplay of multiple factors, 207
leaky gut, 214–217
medications, 210–212
microbiome, 214–217
overview, 204–206
role of thymus gland in aging, 207–208
strategies to counter, 208–214
strategies to help gut health/gut microbiome, 217–221
supplements and herbs, 213–214
Systemic Chronic Inflammation (SCI), 57–59

T

tai chi, 288
tasty toxins, 254–256
T cells, 27
technological tools in mindfulness, 308–309
telomeres, 53, 89, 109
tesamorelin, 198
testosterone, 2, 60, 170, 173–178, 180–182, 184, 201, 236–239, 320, 325
testosterone deficiency, 173–174
testosterone optimization therapy (TOT), 173–178
　estrogen blockers in, 177–178
　gonadorelin in, 178
　human chorionic gonadotropin (HCG) in, 178
　VitalLife approach, 174–175
testosterone replacement therapy (TRT), 174
THC (tetrahydrocannabinol), 263
therapeutic plasma exchange (TPE), 102–104
thiazolidinediones (TZDs), 196
Thiel, Peter, 27
thymic involution, 57, 207
thymosin alpha 1, 198
thymus gland in aging, 207–208
thyroid hormones, 184–185
tissue regeneration, 103
T lymphocytes, 27
traditional healthcare, 9, 15
traditional herbal medicine, 196–197
traditional medicine, 15–18
transcendent mind, 140–142
transformative lifestyle, 40–41
traumatic brain injury (TBI), 123, 160, 165
triggers, 270
trimix, 237
triphala, 294
tumor necrosis factor-alpha (TNF-α), 68, 93
turmeric, 197, 213
Tutu, Bishop Desmond, 33
Twain, Mark, 33
type 2 diabetes, 14, 58, 62, 68–69, 121, 192, 196, 207, 246, 265–266, 278
Tyson, Mike, 149

U

ultra-personalized compounded medications, 222–240
　compounded hormones and peptides, 235–240
　compounded oral ketamine for microdosing protocol, 226–228
　glutathione, 234–235
　intravenous (IV) infusion therapies, 230–232
　low-dose naltrexone (LDN), 228–229
　NAD+, 232–234
　overview, 222–224
　rapamycin, 224–226
　sermorelin, 229–230
unholy trinity, 41, 192, 251–254, 328
Unity Biotechnology, 27

University of California, San Francisco (UCSF), 324
University of Florida College of Medicine, 6
Upanishads, 146
urolithin A, 194, 202, 274, 326
ursolic acid, 202
US Centers for Disease Control and Prevention (CDC), 78
US Drug Enforcement Administration (DEA), 153

V

vascular aging, 74
vegetables-and-fruits-only diet, 261
Venter, Craig, 27
vertebral facet joint area, 130
very-low-dose (VLD) therapy, 166, 227, 325
Vietnam War, 154, 163
Virchow, Rudolf, 76
vitality, 110
VitalLife Aging Triad, 39–40, 67
VitalLife Biomarker Blueprint, 88
VitalLife model of aging, 70–72
VitalLife program, 9–11, 33–43, 115, 173
    benefits of, 36–37
    cellular rejuvenation, 38–39
    chronic inflammation, 39–40
    hormonal optimization, 39
    metabolic insulin resistance, 39–40
    mitochondrial dysfunction, 39–40
    peptide optimization, 39
    personalized assessment/testing, 38
    personalized medicines, 40
    pillars of, 36–41
    regenerative medicine, 38–39
    transformative lifestyle, 40–41
VitalLifeProgram.com, 341

vitamin D_3, 194, 201, 273, 295, 326
vitamin levels, 89
vitamins and nutritional supplements, 201
Volatile Organic Compounds (VOC) testing, 94
Voltaire, 65

W

waist-to-height ratio (WtHR), 90
walking, 287
Wasson, R. Gordon, 144–145
WebMD, 297
weightlifting, 286
weight management, 267
well-being, 156, 171
    emotional, 41, 51, 132, 141, 144, 153, 167, 183–184, 240, 252, 281–285, 289, 302, 308
    holistic, 167
    mental, 51, 166, 216, 285, 302, 310
    optimal, 305
    physical, 285, 310, 315
    psychological, 153
    sense of, 3, 172, 175, 183
wellness drink, 274
Western healthcare system, 13, 16
White Blood Cell (WBC) count, 93
whole-system healing, 151
Woods, Tiger, 115

Y

Yamanaka, Shinya, 97, 118
yoga, 288, 306–307
youthful longevity, 1–11, 23–25
youthfulness and longevity
    action plan for, 319–330
    Aging Triad, 326–327
    biomarker tests for personalized plan, 322–323

hormone and peptide
  optimization, 325–326
lifestyle modifications, 328–330
multifaceted approach for
  maximum impact, 320–322
for people over forty, 322
for people under forty with a
  disease, 322
for people under forty with no
  disease, 321–322
regenerative modalities for cellular
  regeneration, 323–325
special personalized compounded
  medicines, 327–328

Z

zombie cells, 55–56, 104–105
Zuckerberg, Mark, 28

ABOUT THE AUTHOR

Hardesh Garg, MD, affectionately called "Dr. G" by his patients, is a renowned expert in regenerative, anti-aging, and functional medicine. Guided by a simple yet profound personal vision statement, "Improve lives," Dr. G has been a physician for forty years, including twenty years pioneering the fields of regenerative medicine, anti-aging treatments, and functional medicine in the United States. With unmatched expertise, he specializes in anti-aging protocols and cutting-edge regenerative therapies for youthfulness and optimal healthspan.

Patients from across the United States—and from as far as Europe, the Middle East, Asia, and Australia—travel to seek his advanced treatments and personalized protocols. Among his patients are professional athletes from the NFL, NHL, golf, tennis, and other sports, as well as prominent figures who rely on him to optimize their health, performance, and longevity. He continues to help his patients at his VitalLife clinic in Florida (VitalLifeProgram.com)

Dr. G is also a successful serial entrepreneur, clinical researcher, and product innovator. His passion for helping patients extends to developing transformative medicines and technologies for the diseases of aging, with a special focus on improving healthspan. As the founder of VitalLife Pharmaceuticals (VitalLifeProgram.com/pharma), he leads groundbreaking drug development work to address conditions such as atherosclerosis, sarcopenia, traumatic brain injuries, and Alzheimer's disease, among others.

Driven by a deep sense of purpose after his wife, Bina, was diagnosed with schizophrenia, Dr. G cofounded Bina Cares Foundation (Binacares.org) with his wife, a nonprofit organization with the audacious mission to alleviate suffering for families impacted by schizophrenia and other neuropsychiatric brain disorders worldwide.

Dr. G's journey began in India, where he enrolled in a prestigious medical college in New Delhi at the age of seventeen. After completing his medical training and a brief tenure as junior faculty at his alma mater, he immigrated to the United States in 1989. Since then, he has served as clinical assistant professor at the University of Florida College of Medicine and at the University of South Florida College of Medicine. With extensive experience conducting preclinical and human clinical trials, Dr. G has collaborated with international pharmaceutical companies and contributed to clinical research funded by the National Institutes of Health (NIH). A consultant and speaker, he has delivered lectures for global pharmaceutical leaders such as Pfizer, GlaxoSmithKline, and Bristol-Myers Squibb.

Whether caring for patients, guiding clinical research, or through his nonprofit work, Dr. G's calling is unwavering: to transform lives, advance medicine, and bring hope to individuals and families affected by complex health challenges.

www.ingramcontent.com/pod-product-compliance
Lightning Source LLC
Chambersburg PA
CBHW020531030426
42337CB00013B/803